The Waiting Room:
Invisible Voices of Lyme

Stories by

Vickie Gould
Becky Bugala
Elise Bugala
Sam Bugala
Jillian Burgess
Cassidy Colbert
John Coughlin
Lori Dennis
Nancy Fisher
Michael Gould
Rachael Goetz
Jennifer Heath
Carleen Eve Fischer Hoffman
Carole Kamerman
Kim Luton
Stephanie Lyskawa
Candice Mallicoat
Kelsey O'Brien
Laurie Penner
George Popovici
Niki Slovacek
Alana Stamper
Shelley White
Jenna Wright

DISCLAIMER

This book is not intended to diagnose, treat, cure or prevent any disease. This book is not intended as medical advice. This book is only intended to share personal experiences. This book is provided for informational and educational purposes only, not as a treatment guide or instructions for any disease.

Many disease are serious and requires the treatment of a licensed physician. This book is not to be used to substitute for professional medical care. Do not begin any new treatment program without full consent and supervision from a licensed physician. If you have a medical problem, consult a doctor, not this book. If you are pregnant or breastfeeding, consult a doctor before using any treatment.

Vickie Gould offers no guarantee that the ideas in this book are the best therapies for your condition(s). They are simply ideas that the authors inside this anthology felt compelled to write about. Do not rely on this book as final treatment in any condition however mild or severe.

DEDICATION

To all those who have suffered and continue to suffer with Lyme Disease. You are not alone.

And to my beautiful friend Che Chin Lie (12/21/77 - 9/17/15) who was a light for so many with Lyme.

Table of Contents

STORIES FROM CAREGIVERS

ACKNOWLEDGMENTS

Thank you to each author in this book who was willing to contribute their story to spread Lyme awareness. It's not easy to share our innermost thoughts and personal experiences and I commend you for being willing to put yourself out there for the sake of helping others.

Wondering

By Vickie Gould

It's the thoughts I had that I never wanted to tell anyone. I didn't really want to die. I just wanted to stop living THIS WAY. What would they think if I admitted it? What would happen if they knew? Would they think I was making too much out of nothing and being over dramatic? Would I be seen as weak? What would my husband think? What about the kids, if they ever found out?

I didn't want to have a handgun in the house. I knew what would happen if I knew how to load and use it. And I hated that I even had any thoughts about it at all.

It just felt like everyone would be better off without me here, including me. I was a drain on the family's finances, I couldn't even get up to make the kids lunch in the mornings before school. I had a hard time cleaning, doing laundry or cooking dinner. I couldn't remember where I was going in the car or what I was doing half-way through a task.

I didn't have the energy to be a mom or a wife.

An "acquaintance-friend" even reprimanded me for wearing my PJ's to Walmart. Was that really disgraceful? I had my coat on ….

And every day started the same. I'd wake up exhausted, disappointed that the light was peaking through the sides of the black-out curtains already. Even though I wanted to sleep, it eluded me most nights. How in the world could someone be so tired and yet not be able to sleep?

I immediately started wishing for nighttime to come again, wondering when in the day I could go back to bed. I laid there few more moments giving myself a pep talk about the day before rolling over, sitting up, and dangling my feet off the side of the bed. I looked down at the floor and wondered what my body would feel once my feet hit the carpet and I stood up, full weight on them.

"Wondering," was what happened a lot with Lyme

Disease.

I wondered how long I would last in the day.
I wondered if I could make it to my doctor's
appointments.
I wondered if I could finish more than 1 task per day.
I wondered what my children would grow up with as
their memories of their mom.
I wondered if the next treatment would help (or even be
the one that "fixed" me).
I wondered who I was anymore.

And I wondered how many more days I could endure
the physical pain, the emotional pain, the feelings of
uselessness and failure.

Plus there were all the regrets about what I had not yet
been able to do in life.

I wondered if I would ever get to do them, and the idea
that "never" was the answer gave me an agony inside
like I was screaming and crying all at the same time, in
a small ball in the corner inside myself where no one

else could hear.

The real truth of the matter is, "You don't get it until you get it," with Lyme Disease. The symptoms list is long – pain and widespread inflammation, migraines, blurred vision, attention deficit, dyslexia, dementia, digestion issues, cognitive disorder, arthritis, muscle spasms, depression, anxiety, depersonalization, hormonal imbalances, chemical sensitivities, noise sensitivities, vertigo …. I've seen lists that share hundreds of symptoms and labels (including mis-labels) that Lyme disease carries.

Lyme never comes to the party alone. It's way more complex than that. It's the coinfections, gene mutations, mold issues and chemical imbalances, amongst other things, that create such a misunderstood disease which gets misdiagnosed all too often - and poor testing doesn't help either. It's like chasing your tail and never catching it. And as soon as you find out one thing, there's another to complicate it all.

It's hard to explain because it's invisible. Think about it

this way: EVERYTHING is inflamed, including your brain and everything is amplified, making you super sensitive. Merely going out can be frightening.

The Grocery Store

I couldn't drive further than a few minutes from my home. When we moved just 5 minutes away from the grocery store, I was so relieved. Problem was the grocery store parking lot was huge and the grocery store itself seemed monstrous.

As I drove up to the red bricked Meijer grocery store, I started to get that sinking feeling. Where will I park? Will I even remember where I parked? I needed to park in the same area I usually do so I won't forget.

Often times as the glass automatic double doors opened to let me out, I wouldn't know where to go and thought my car had been stolen. My heart would start to race, my eyes would pan the parking lot in panic and I tried not to let anyone see that I was lost. I desperately hoped I wouldn't need to call my husband.

But what had just happened inside only added to my stress. Even though I'd used a list to get the groceries, inevitably, I would forget something that was in the opposite corner of the mega grocery store. It would just about bring me to tears to think about walking back to get the item.

I looked around the brightly lit store, the fresh veggies on the right, clothing to the left and the pharmacy even further to the left. Did I really need to go over there? Could we live without the item I had on the list? I hoped no one who saw me could see I was on the brink of tears. My body hurt, my mind was foggy, pushing the weight of the cart was using up all the energy I had for the day and I still had other things that had to happen.

I had to decide. Yes or no? Do I get the item or not?

I would've loved to have the option to order the groceries for curbside pickup as they do now. That would've been so nice! But guess what? A Lyme friend actually said that someone told her that using that service meant she was lazy. What kind of friend is that?

The Doctor's Office

When I got the diagnosis of chronic Lyme Disease I thought it was a happy moment. I thought it meant there was a protocol.   I thought that I could kick out my misdiagnosis of Lupus, early onset osteoarthritis and early onset perimenopause.

I thought wrong.

The doctors weren't sure what to do with me. I blindly followed the advice of taking antibiotics and did seven months of them. It felt like they were killing me and they literally were killing my guts.

After those seven months, I couldn't take it anymore so I decided to go the natural route and got a rife machine and used a lot of herbs. I did so much research, I think Google was the best friend I talked to the most. In the course of 3.5 years, I tried a lot of things – from protocols meant for malaria to ingesting food grade hydrogen peroxide, LDA and rifing, sauna, dry brushing, etc … I threw everything I could at it. Many times the treatment made me feel worse.

And I'd drive up to see my next Lyme doctor and get IV treatments, but the problem was that the 30 minute drive there and then the 30 minute drive back home did me in for about a week afterwards. About the time I would recover, it'd be time to go back again.

So when the doctor asked me if I could feel a difference, I told him I couldn't tell because the driving was probably negating any of the benefits of the IV. Even he didn't believe me - my own Lyme doctor, of all people should believe me, right?

Of course social security didn't believe me either. I fought to get the help I needed twice over the course of those years. The first time, I trusted the lawyer too much and wasted a lot of time. The judge even threw out my medical records. How does that even make sense? Eventually, I got it, but it was not for Lyme as it's not recognized. I got it for fibromyalgia.

My Husband and Kids

I think one of the worst effects of Lyme is what it does to families. I was angry for so many reasons, and on top if it, had what they call "Lyme Rage."

Remember how I said everything was inflamed, including the brain? Well everything – every body system is invaded by bacteria spirochetes called Lyme. It's neurological, cardiovascular, muscular-skeletal – it's everywhere. They take over the communication system. Release horrible toxins into your body and disrupt the chemical and hormonal balances inside as well. They take over the communication systems inside you too. They hide in joints, burrow into your brain and spinal column, and your little white blood cell soldiers are duped and walk on by.

Anger got the best of me.

I was angry because my husband had taken me camping way too many times. I blamed him for my going outside and getting sick. I had gone camping for him.

I was angry that I had to depend on someone and constantly ask for help when I was used to being the Superwoman that everyone else asked to help them.

I was angry that I couldn't go to my children's field trips or their school parties. They were too draining and over stimulating. Plus if they were outdoors ….

I was angry that my child needed me to fill a sippy cup when I couldn't get off the couch.

I was angry that dirt and dust accumulated on the floor and the toilets had to be cleaned.

I was angry that it was morning already and I never felt refreshed.

And I took it out on everyone around me.

Little things set me off. I would scream at the top of my

lungs at the kids. I would argue with my husband and as I would yell, cry and spew my venom, inside my head I would say to myself, "Stop it. Why are you yelling? They didn't really even do anything that big. Can't you just stop?"

But I couldn't stop. It was like I was watching myself outside of myself and I couldn't control it. I just kept going.

And eventually some days, I made my husband cry. In an odd, warped way, that satisfied me. I wanted him to feel as bad as I felt because some days he made me feel bad. I blamed him for going camping over and over again. I felt like he didn't support me. He yelled at me the day I asked for help with the laundry, "Well, if I have to do that too, I might as well quit my job!" He didn't understand what was going on with me and I thought he should try harder to understand.

I started to call him my fair-weathered husband and one day I took all his clothes out of the closet and dumped them on the floor. I really wanted to throw them all on the front lawn or out the back window. What kind of man acts like they can't take it anymore and wants to walk away?

What I didn't understand was that he was grieving the woman he had married. She was not the same.

Honestly, what I wanted to do many days was to take all the dishes and throw them at a tree just to watch them smash into smithereens. I wanted an outlet for this rage. But I also didn't have the energy for it.

Could I be THAT mom?

I could tell I was getting better. The rollercoaster of flares was getting more manageable. The string of bad days were getting shorter and the string of good days were getting longer. Could it really be that the switch might be flipping? Yet there was a plateau of wellness I couldn't get past. I had tried just about everything.

Everything but ONE thing – cannabis.

I wondered …. Could I be that mom? I didn't want to be THAT mom – the mom that was high all day.

All my life I had been against drugs. I had taught my children the same.

But during the time I researched all those herbs, I also became a Master Herbalist, and I came to realize that just like Lyme, cannabis was very misunderstood.

It took me almost a year to "cave in" to my thoughts on what kind of example this would be if my kids found out. I did it the legal way and got my card. The first couple of strains were not the right ones for sure! But eventually, I found what worked – a high THC that actually didn't make me high. It just helped me sleep.

Cannabis put me over that last plateau and gave me my life back. I fought Lyme, coinfections, MTHFR, hormone imbalances, mold (sick building syndrome) and so much inside my mind.

Belief

While I was going through the worst parts of my Lyme journey, people said such silly things....

"You just need to exercise more."
"You just need to get out and be social more."
"You just need to eat _____."

Or the lovely, "I have such-and-such symptom too." Uh .... Are you for real? Would you ever tell a cancer patient you had their same symptoms? I think not.

The one thing I will say helped a lot was actually being able to sleep – it's the natural restorative process your body needs every day. In fact, my Lyme doctor told me, "If you do not figure out a way to actually get some sleep, you will never get better." I took that to heart.

And I had to also figure out how to get my body to detox. Between my MTHFR gene mutation and the mold that was backed up in my system, Lyme had an easy time taking hold of me.

When people said things like, "Just think positively," it just made me more angry and irritated that they could even suggest it was that simple. You try to think positively when you're going through the darkest moments of your life alone! On the other hand, I do believe that letting go of the idea that I was destined to live a slow and painful death and that nothing would get better helped me tremendously.

When I decided that I was going to get better and I wouldn't accept a prognosis of "forever" and "incurable," THAT was when I thought less and less about the handgun I couldn't have in the house or the garden tub in which I could drown myself.

It was the BELIEF that my life was meant for more and that this Lyme journey was meant for something that got me through. At the time, I didn't know what that something was.

Today, I believe it's so that I could live out the life I had imagined in my head but had always denied myself. It was about those regrets I thought about all day and night – it was time to make those happen! I also believe that I went through this Lyme journey so that I could encourage people not to give up and I could help people see that little faint light at the end of the tunnel called, "Hope."

Bridges

by Jenna Wright

As I began to recover enough from my Lyme and Complex Illness experience, I ventured out again, in 2013, to our annual vacation on Sanibel Island. But, this particular year, the Sanibel Taxi Company met me at the marina, before the causeway, with an extra driver, to escort me and my daughter, in our auto, over the causeway.

My brain had not yet repaired enough from the encephalopathy that caused myriad vision issues, including improper depth perception and very choppy transition from peripheral to tunnel vision. My vision was much better, but not enough to fully trust the communication between my brain and visual perceptions. The bridge, the potential for misjudgment by my eyes, was a safety concern for me.

People thought I was crazy, including some family members, and they simply couldn't grasp that I could have an issue driving over a bridge. They either chalked it up to a phobia and rolled their eyes at me or suggested I should stay home, heal more and wait another year. But, that didn't matter one bit to me. I was going to get over that bridge today!

As I looked back at my illness, the greatest moments of self-centeredness arrived within my experience of Lyme Disease. An illness, so traumatic in its onset, that I could barely see, feel and hear anything outside of one foot from my self. A 24/7 roller coaster ride through hell with one foot, dragging, digging my grave, into which, I fought continually to avoid falling. Everyday lives went on around me while a bombastic war was occurring within me. Doctors and family would speak and my mind would inaccurately translate their foreign language, me responding, at times, with my backwards nonsensical English, while my mind shouted "Shut up! Just Please Shut Up!!! Can't you see the hell I'm in?! Do something! Help me! I AM DYING, DAMMIT !!!"

Daily waves of Death's grip, tugging, pulling and me breathing through, resisting, while someone talked about their kids grades, college, a new recipe, telling me "you'll feel better after a shower and some makeup".....all received in my mind as benign bullshit.

And I'd scream, again, inside my head "I can't tolerate your words...you really don't get it...can't you see! Why can't you see the terror in my eyes and that I, my whole being, body/mind/soul, is in shock. I'm a zombie with a palpitating, racing heart and brain swelling out of its skeletal container!! What the hell is wrong with you people!!! NO! Going for a walk and socializing won't help me...not when I don't have the mitochondrial energy to put my hands above my head and wash my hair, not when I can't feel all of my legs and they won't stop shaking! Not when I'm so contracted in a pained body that feels like it's going to simultaneously implode and explode. Not when my arms and legs are crossed, hugging myself, clinging as tightly as possible to life. Don't you get that I can't walk in the fetal position!"

My mind would rant at them and what would come out of my mouth in response, with as much energy as I could conjure, in a forced exhausted loud whisper was a simple "Okay". And, I saw that there was no way they could begin to sympathize, much less empathize with my experience, because, this was an epidemic too new, too unbelievably bizarre in all of its symptoms and too traumatic, too ugly, to scary for any of them to understand. An epidemic that touches the whole of the being and may likely be named something entirely different as time and science move along. The closest anyone in my life ever came to "getting it" was when my doctor said that my body was so toxic that it was as if I were receiving 3 high dose chemo treatments per week and that adrenaline was the only thing driving my body.

(A Whole Foods cashier once asked if I was fighting cancer. "Yes" almost came out of my mouth in a manipulative selfish attempt to see empathy in her eyes and maybe get a little human touch with a pat on my hand, because, I knew that people were kind to cancer patients...I wanted some of that kindness)

But, that doctor's description was only a small glimpse of the myriad hells I was experiencing. So many organ systems were involved and all were crashing, tick transmitted viruses that are much like malaria were attacking my body, symptoms of encephalitis were a constant, my liver wasn't filtering, causing all of my body to be bathed in toxins as if I had been poisoned, the scent of chemicals and mold were more than my body could process, light was my enemy and too painful for my eyes to take in, one colitis attack after another and my nights were filled with heart pounding night terrors that would begin the moment I drifted into a fake sleep, sweating, shaking, jerking…anything but sleeping, shoulders frozen and tendons torturously tightened…and many more symptoms too lengthy and ugly to continue describing.

So you see, after all that, I was definitely going across that bridge! I was no longer bed bound, I was upright and ready. I couldn't wait to reach that gulf coast! I felt like a Phoenix rising by making this trip to my favorite place, where I had been every summer for over three decades. I had to celebrate my triumph over death and the bed in which I fought, surrendered and began to recover.

At first, I was disappointed in their lack of understanding, of their inability to grasp the magnitude of what I was experiencing. I wanted them to be joyous with me. To me, this was like a parade level event... a monumental moment. I wanted them to help me figure out a way to get over that bridge and onto my happy little island escape where nothing bad had ever happened and where the past remains behind in the crossing of the causeway and time slows for all of the moments of my week.

The disappointment was fleeting. I quickly went back to the grateful thoughts I had leaned into over the past year... words I would repeat in my head when I felt alone, in an abyss, with no champion...words that would lift me out of my victim mindset and into a space of truth in love...

"It's okay, Jenna. Be happy they can't begin to comprehend. Fully understanding would , require they suffer. This is a complex and traumatic an illness that I would never want them to experience, because, I love them. And, because I love them, I accept their lack of demonstrative compassion with a grateful heart. I am happy that they can't understand"

Then, unexpected compassion came when I called the taxi company. Just 5 minutes before, the owner had watched the national news, releasing the CDC's estimates of 300k new #lymedisease cases per year. I briefly explained my situation and she interrupted me, saying she just saw the news accounts of what I'd experienced. She called it horrific and told me not to worry, that she would have a driver for me and it would be at no charge. Neither she nor anyone she was close to had ever experienced a TBD (tick born disease). Pure compassion...Love in action!

At some point in my months long space and time blurring surreal experience, in the more critical stages of this illness, I began to see inward. I allowed myself to float in this Dali and Kafkaesque experience as it arrived in waves. I flowed with it, into myself. Not in self-centered pain, not in the physical, but truly into myself, my being, my soul the "I Am" of me.

There, I found compassion for those who couldn't "get it", who couldn't see my suffering, either because their soul's eyes had not matured enough or because I had become so adept in my lifetime behavioral training at pretending all was well, with a smile on my face, my lipstick on and the collective memorized, robotic word "Finethankyouandhowareyou?" rolling over my forced smiling lips.

I forgave them because I loved them. And because I loved them, I would not want them to empathetically understand as that would mean they would have to join me in my hells. Who would want someone they love to experience any kind of hell?

So, in the "I Am" of me, I found me. I held me, rocked me, hugged me, and loved me....for the first time in my life. I brushed the hair from my eyes and promised to take care of me, and I assured me that no matter the outcome, all would be okay. Forgiveness, answers, a broadened view beyond my one foot of vision from selfishness that was born in my pain, appeared. I forgave them all.

And Love stayed. In my life before Lyme, it had frequently left, sometimes abruptly, but this time, Love stayed because it came from an eternal source within me. I didn't have to jump through hoops to get it and then bust my ass to keep it happy and hope it remained.

All I had to do was open the door into I AM. Loving me was the key that unlocked it all...healing, peace, confidence, contentment and selflessness....a Treasure Chest of Love's gifts.

When I recognized that my experience with Lyme Disease, while a traumatically consuming epidemic that will prove to have significant implications in the medical, social and spiritual history of mankind, was in fact, NOT the biggest event in the history of the universe, I became able to put it into purposeful perspective.

My end conclusion was that it was merely an event. A powerful event, a surreal and very painful event, but, nonetheless, factually and simply, an event. I saw that in the end, it was the growing and learning and becoming within the event that would prove to be a small part of the largest impact on the history of mankind, if....if, I chose to allow my purpose, my contribution within this impact.

Ultimately, it came down to the simple lesson, for me, to choose to Be Love in all things, surrendering and allowing all purposes their unfolding.

Protocols, in my opinion, are needed stabilizing practicalities. It's the other two thirds of our being that, when allowed to heal, carry us through recovery and fuels the desire to never return to "normal".

A few things I learned during my Lyme health crashes:

I am whole, perfectly made and beautifully unique.

I don't have to own anyone's experience but my own.

I choose. In every moment of every day, I own the power of choice.

I need no approval.

I matter, but, it's not all about me.

I am part of something bigger than any disease or any circumstance and I don't need to know what or why.

I cannot simultaneous sit in judgment against myself or any other person and experience love.

And, most importantly and quite simply…

I am Love.

I have come to have a true belief in my worth, with love for myself, with an understanding that all of my choices in every thought, breath and movement rippled beyond myself and with the awareness that it all had very little to do with only me.

And, I've come to appreciate the function of bridges, both literally and figuratively. Bridges into myself, bridges into others, bridges into God, bridges into truth and the bridge that takes me to my precious paradise, Sanibel Island.

Jenna Wright is an International Functional Health Coach. She has worked in this arena for 16 years. She left employment in the administrative side of the Conventional Medical world, as personal health issues forced her to seek answers to her mysterious illnesses. Answers that no specialists had been able to provide. Her healing and training was found in Functional Medicine, where the best of all healing modalities are used to treat the root causes of illness, rather than the symptoms. She serves as a guide to medical professionals and their patients, assisting them through the mazes in which she once circled.

An internet search of "Jenna Wright Basically Well" will take you to her website and various social media pages.

Nancy Fisher's Lyme Story

By Nancy Fisher

In the winter of 2009-2010, at the age of 45, I fell mysteriously ill with a myriad of symptoms I initially thought were completely disconnected—unprecedented fatigue, 'drop attacks'; i.e., fainting, GI and urinary issues, uncharacteristic irritability, an inability to find words, stammering (from someone who was previously very articulate), etc. Because I was seemingly healthy up to that point, this was a very bizarre turn of events and I pursued treatment, initially with my family doc. and then eventually a series of specialists trying to pinpoint the cause of my symptoms. Little did I know at the outset that my journey had only just begun and that there were no simple answers or even a quick fix to my troubles. I was farmed out from specialist to specialist and had everything from a colonoscopy (which scared the bejeezes out of me since my doc. was trying to rule out colon cancer) to a lower GI and visits with various specialists that pretty much ran the gamut—two immunologists, a toxicologist, a neurologist, a hematologist, a pulmonologist, an environmental medicine doc., a naturopath and several other 'alternative' practitioners.

One of the hallmarks of my new illness seemed to be the development of exquisite environmental sensitivities which was only heightened when my employer replaced some carpeting in the office kitchen, a relatively small room and down the hall from where I sat. The fact that I was the only person in my small firm to become so sickened and sensitized was not lost on me but I still didn't know what to make of it. I just knew it was real. I had to step away from that job and did not attempt to return to work until several months later at which time I began reacting to the very strong perfume of one of my new co-workers. Another job lost and no closer to having an answer as to WHY!

A few months later, we were chatting about this strange and mystifying turn of events with a friend when she said, "You sound just like my friend and her Mom (both of whom lived in New York) who have Lyme Disease". She was the second person to mention Lyme Disease and so my ears perked up and I listened intently. I eventually made my way to a Lyme-literate medical doctor (LLMD) who clinically diagnosed me with Chronic Lyme Disease and even linked my extreme chemical sensitivities to Lyme. Based on my bloodwork (I had very, very low white blood cells), he guestimated that I had likely contracted Lyme Disease as a child and had perhaps even been recently reinfected—which is very plausible given the fact that just six months prior hubby and I had been hiking in the Finger Lakes region of New York, a VERY Lyme-endemic region. I'm of Norwegian heritage and the woods are my cathedral. I was a tomboy growing up and spent my summers up North hanging out with a lot of my brother's friends in the woods and on the beach or at the lake. While I don't recall ever seeing a tick on me or even having the telltale bulls eye rash (I've since learned not everyone gets the rash or it can be in places that are not very visible), my risk potential for Lyme is HUGE. If there was a wooded glen, you'd find me in it and as an adult, my vacations were really hiking trips loosely organized around farm-to-table restaurants, my two great loves.

The LLMD I saw prescribed prescription antibiotics and

systemic antifungals, neither of which I was comfortable with and I knew intuitively that it was not the strategy I wanted to pursue. As someone who was previously very proud and independent, I was extremely depressed (devastated really) that I was unable to work and support myself; I spent most of my days lying in bed crying, literally all day. Looking back, I can now see that I was severely cognitively impacted and that was only worsened by the periodic environmental exposures to things like fragrance, commercial cleaners, gasoline, synthetic chemicals of every kind, etc. I came to realize that I had a 'leaky brain' which often occurs in chronically ill people where chemicals and pathogens gain access to your brain, an area that if you are healthy, is generally off limits to these invaders. At this point, I saw my chemical sensitivities as my biggest hurdle and chose to see an out-of-state specialist who treated people with neurological issues caused by chemical exposures. Sometimes the Universe leads you to the resources you need and this was one example. This Angel masquerading as a doctor placed me on a protocol that partially brought me back from the walking dead and that restored a bit of hope. Things were not perfect and I was still fairly reactive to my environment but for the first time I felt like maybe there was a light at the end of the tunnel … and that for a change it wasn't an oncoming train!

A few months later, I found a Lyme-literate Naturopathic doc. (LLND) in Vermont and we made the arduous 13-hour drive from Michigan to Vermont, popping supplements and nebulizing compounds all the while as I drove (with hubby as my able nursing assistant). I took Lyme herbals for about six months but quite honestly did not feel like it made much of a dent in my symptoms. However, when I felt like giving up, my hubby became my cheerleader, singlehandedly working to support the both of us to pay my ever-mounting out-of-pocket medical expenses (the herbal, more holistic treatments I opted to pursue were not covered by insurance and were completely out-of-pocket). My environmental sensitivities seemed to worsen and I kept researching and reading (to the extent that I could cognitively grasp things), hoping to find an answer.

In 2014, I came across the work of Ritchie Shoemaker,

M.D. who pioneered the medical treatment of mold illness. While there were some symptoms that fit, I wasn't sure that this was going to turn out to be my problem. However, when I got to a local Shoemaker doctor, I discovered that I was genetically susceptible for both Lyme Disease and mold illness, one of the 1-2% of the general population for whom that is true. I laughingly joke that I lost the genetic lotto. My lab markers were also very positive for mold/biotoxin illness or CIRS (Chronic Inflammatory Response Syndrome). In retrospect, I can look back—with 20/20 vision—and realized that the myriad of symptoms I had when I lived in a moldy tri-level many moons ago were classic for mold illness and that a later, almost 1-year sabbatical on the North Coast of California, was very indicative of mold exposure (our apartment at the time had visible mold).

What I want to say to anyone who has Lyme Disease is that it is often not JUST the Lyme Disease that made you ill although it's understandably tempting to focus all your efforts on Lyme. It's all about your biological terrain which is really what effects your body's ability to fight off the bugs, whether that's Lyme or its co-infections. I didn't understand that initially and as I peel this onion, it's sometimes only in retrospect that I can look back and see how various insults weakened my system and made me susceptible to getting so sick, even though it felt like I lost my health almost overnight. Hindsight, as they say, is 20/20. That is still a process and I know there are other facets of my health challenges that I have yet to identify and address before I will be able to fully recover. The year 2016 was one of transition. I recently looked back at the Treatment Record that I maintain and was blown away by how many simultaneous holistic treatments I was pursuing at that time. However, that was likely responsible for moving the needle to the point where my crippling chemical sensitivities lessened considerably. They haven't resolved completely and I have to watch what I expose myself to but I can now go out in public and be exposed to people who are wearing moderate amounts of fragrance and/or who are walking around in a cloud of dryer sheet residue without being immediately stupefied and incapable of speaking or even functioning. I'm still not back to work and I have a LOT of work to go but for the first time in 7 years, I feel like I have a stronger conceptual framework for what I'm dealing with and what the roadmap to wellness looks like. I am currently working with a couple of different holistic practitioners to address different facets of my health as I continue to peel the onion.

I can honestly say that as soul sucking as this whole experience has been, it has been my greatest life lesson. I've gone from someone who had a very black and white perspective on life to someone who is willing to dabble with a palette of greys. And perhaps one of my greatest lessons has been to practice compassion, both toward others and toward myself.

They've Stopped Asking
by Rachael Goetz

It's 12:03 A.M. and I am so exhausted but can't sleep.
My hands and feet have decided to swell to twice their
size & feel like they are 100 degrees, all while the rest
of my body is freezing cold. My heart is thumping in my
chest, I feel as if there is a complete sheet of wax paper
over my left eye, and my blood pressure has dropped
because the dizziness and fogginess is heading in.

These symptoms used to send us flying to the ER,
where they would stare at me perplexed for several
hours and then send us home without having even
touched me. Thankfully this is my 6th year in this
journey of Lyme Disease and I have learned a lot.

This would be Lyme rearing its ugly head again
because as a busy mama of 4 littles I have once again
done too much or stressed a little too much, or maybe
those Dove Chocolates called my name and I will pay
for each sweet heart I have eaten! My diagnosis didn't
come easily. I fought, cried and begged for every

specialist appointment, blood test, procedure, and diagnosis. 35 doctors, 3 big hospitals, and four 4 inch binders of medical documents. Praise God because as I was literally losing the ability to walk, talk, drive, and was wondering if I would be alive to see Christmas with my sweet children who were 6,3,3, and 12 months at the time.

At the last hour, an internist who thinks outside the box tested me with a specialized Igenex Lyme Disease test and I tested positive. After fighting 3 long years, this diagnosis was accompanied with joy, tears, and relief. However, the journey had just started.

Many do not believe Chronic Lyme disease exists and explaining it to friends and family often brought tears and frustration as they looked at you like I was a cat from the wrong side of the tracks as I explained everything!

I am 6 years into this disease and there are good days & bad days. People have stopped asking how you feel because after 6 years, you must be well?!?! Plus, you look so cute in your new pair of leggings and sweater boots, that you have to be all better, right?!?!

I simply smile and respond that there are good days & bad days. On bad days I have more ailments than an 80 year old lady! Six months of cold weather drills deep into my muscles, joints and soul. The pain comes back and the ability to use my hands, braid my daughters hair, and truck through the simple tasks of the day become a luxury.

But on good days I can grocery shop (something I was so happy to get back to), cook dinner, tidy the house, volunteer at school, and also help my littles with homework. The good days are so good and they are the days I sing God praises. This disease take a lot out of a marriage, relationships with family and friends, and others who just don't get it.

But, I am grateful for my tribe, for the people who still ask, for my amazing husband who can take one look at my eyes and says, "You need to go lay down right now, for my parents who still help in every way possible, and for my sister who 6 years later still calls every single morning to see how I am feeling, and most of all I am grateful that I am still alive and slowly making improvements.

I have never given up on any challenge and don't intend to now! Lyme Disease is something I wouldn't wish on my worst enemy, but I will share my journey to educate others and fight with all I have because my family and my dreams are way too important to let Lyme Disease take them away.

Amazing Results: The Healing Power of Cannabis Oil on Lyme Disease and Co-Infections

By Shelley M. White

The beginning of my journey with Lyme disease is similar to most. My ending, however, is playing out quite differently than most. I found a tick behind my ear at the age of fourteen, and had various health problems for seven years before I was finally diagnosed with Lyme disease, Lupus, Mycoplasma, Bartonella, and Babesia. After two years my Lupus, Mycoplasma, Bartonella and Babesia are entirely eradicated. As far as my Lyme disease goes, I now have zero symptoms. My remaining ones are a result of withdrawals from the prescriptions I so naively started taking when I was initially diagnosed.

How am I already returning to a healthy lifestyle only two years after forgetting to read, write, walk and talk? Well, a wealth of credit is owed to the Buhner protocol. I would not be where I am today without it. Still, I had one last giant "hump" in healing to get over after a year on the protocol. So I took a shot in the dark which, for me, turned out to be the path to light. I decided to make my own cannabis oil and began taking it every waking hour. I now owe my life to this fascinating herb and am hopeful some of you will find strength and encouragement through this information.

For a year and a half I had over ten seizures a day. I tried every treatment I could find, exhausting outlets in both conventional and holistic medicine. Desperately searching for answers, I stumbled across what turned out to be one of the most profound facts I have ever learned. Marijuana contains one of the most potent anticonvulsants in the world. Controversy over the subject was meaningless at that point, as the herb offered a possible solution to one of my most debilitating symptoms. As it turned out, smoking marijuana not only controlled my seizures, it completely cured them. With that in mind, I moved forward with my research. If it could do for seizures what no other plant or prescription could do, what could it do for Lyme? What I found was nothing short of fascinating, and essentially lifesaving.

Cannabis has over 700 healing components which, to the best of my knowledge, is more than any other plant known to mankind. Since my Lyme disease had reacted to and benefited from literally every herb I had taken, I figured it would without a doubt react to cannabis as well. Indeed, it did. Smoking marijuana had sometimes made me feel sick in the past, and I realized this could possibly be because it caused a Herxheimer reaction from bacteria die off each time. Experimenting what thankfully turned out to be an anything but crazy theory, I smoked an exceptionally large amount one night and suffered from a massive Herxheimer reaction. The next day, when it subsided, I felt I had regained a little chunk of my brain back. Since smoking the herb out of a regular pipe also means inhaling a lot of toxins, I began using a vaporizer to get more cannaniboids. My rate of improvement significantly sped up when I did this. Naturally, this motivated me to take treatment one step further and find out what the results of taking cannabis oil would do for me. After only a month of taking it I was able to return to work and school, and began to drive and have a social life again. Now, I am finally planning to move out and be independent for the first time in years. Basically, I am returning to a lifestyle that I was once unsure I would ever see again thanks to the immense healing power of cannabis oil.

Understandably, some will negate this story due to preconceived notions regarding cannabis, ones we were all conditioned to believe from a young age. Even I once held strong beliefs that cannabis was harmful to my health, but I could not be more thankful that I was proven otherwise. For me, the tangible proof stemming from first-hand experience will always trump the mere words of others.

Please browse through the CE website to find more links about the medicinal benefits of this herb. You can start here and here.

No Bullseye

by Kim Luton

I was officially diagnosed with Lyme in April 2016 but I believe my Lyme journey started at least four years earlier during a vacation to see family in Southern Illinois. I had no bullseye rash but attributed the symptoms I was experiencing to thyroid disease which I have lived with for at least 15 years. I experienced lethargy, brain fog, loss of memory, unexplained weight gain and my joints ached all the time, particularly in my right hip and right knee.

Prior to diagnosis, and given I prefer a holistic method of medical treatment to conventional Western medicine, I began Chiropractic and massage care thinking that would improve my mobility. I began changing my eating habits cutting out as much sugar as possible as studies I read indicated sugar fueled some of the symptoms I had. I researched essential oils and began incorporating them into my care.

Then in April, 2016 my right knee swelled all the way to

my ankle for no reason. My orthopedic doctor recognized that I was experiencing either gout or Lyme disease. He took samples of my synovial fluid and the results came back positive for Lyme. He was so sure it was Lyme, he immediately started me on a 30 day course of antibiotics. The antibiotics did reduce the swelling but I had Lyme for much longer and damage had already been done to my joints. As soon as I completed the antibiotic treatment, I started probiotics to rebuild my gut.

I was fortunate to run into a friend who told me about a doctor who was having success with patients by treating Lyme and co-infections with radio-frequency. I had a friend who bought a RIFE machine and was self-treating for Lyme with success so my mind was very open to alternative medicine. My first treatment was five hours and I was tested for borrellia and many co-infections. I experienced a lot of herxing for the next several days. I have had several more treatments since the bacteria seems to have a life cycle but my life is much improved. Damage to my joints is permanent but I am managing with massage and essential oils.

I know I have been very fortunate in comparison to others who have had much worse symptoms for long term. I believe now that some of the symptoms I was attributing to thyroid disease were actually Lyme. I am very thankful for my doctor, Dr. Rich Price, who I attribute my wellness to as well as my massage therapist who helped me with my mobility.

Kim Luton, Dover, DE

Focusing on Just Me

By Anonymous

My Lyme story started in 2012. I had been experiencing increasing pain in multiple joints. This was puzzling to both my doctor and me as I was pretty active and hit the gym almost every day of the week. After several months, the pain became so bad that I stopped working out. I had difficulty walking and using my hands. I felt like I had aged 20 years.

I consulted with a rheumatologist, a doctor who was well recognized at a local teaching hospital. He diagnosed me with atypical rheumatoid arthritis, atypical because all the tests were negative. He prescribed prednisone to manage joint swelling and pain, and an immunosuppressant to manage the arthritis. Little did I know that even with all this doctor's wisdom and significant credentials, his actions set the stage for a massive decline in health that would impact both my personal and professional life.

About a week into treatment, I contacted the doctor's

office. I was feeling horrible and the pain was worse. His administrative assistant responded and said not to worry, it would take time for medication to work and I should continue taking the medication.

The following weekend was a holiday. I was miserable. By Sunday, I had broken out in weird rashes all over my body. Some of the rashes were round, and some were stripes. I called the doctor's office and spoke to the covering physician. After listening to my story, she suggested that the round rashes might be the Lyme EM rash and recommended Lyme testing. She was right. The Lyme test was positive. The rheumatologist prescribed 2 weeks of antibiotics. When I finished the prescribed course, he said I was cured, although I felt no better. He said that it was "Post Lyme Syndrome" and I would just have to work through it.

In tears, I returned to my primary, who is an integrative physician. He apologized for missing the Lyme and started me on multiple antibiotics following the Horowitz protocol. We also added multiple alternative treatments, especially focusing on detoxification. He recommended lots of rest. He said recovery would be long and we would work together. He set the expectation that we would need to tweek our approach regularly to stay on top of issues as things cropped up. We did coinfection testing and found multiple issues that we needed to address. In retrospect, those striped rashes that I saw while working with the rheumatologist was probably Bartonella!

He also recommended genetic testing to rule out metabolic issues. After months of antibiotic treatment, my liver couldn't keep up with the detox. I had to discontinue antibiotics which pushed me into the world of herbal and homeopathic treatment

While this was happening, my employer was being uncooperative. They wanted me in the office although my doctor said to work from home. They required weekly reports from my doctor which became a huge burden for him.

They forced me to take short term disability instead of working from home. When I ran out of Short Term Disability, they made me apply for Long Term Disability, which was denied at which point they terminated my employment. I was shattered as I had been a hard worker for this company for 8 years.

Eventually, I grew to realize that this was probably the best thing that could have happened. I gave myself time to grieve the loss of my job and to be angry about both the illness and my ex-employer. My husband was really supportive and told me to just focus on me. Having been in high tech industry for decades, we have gone through being on a single income before. We have also both had health issues before, so he understood how much work it takes to get ones health back on track.

Former co-workers reached out. They were horrified to hear what had happened and to learn what I had been going through with my health. Their kindness and support helped me with the pain of letting go of my previous job. I missed those that I was friends with, but I knew that I would stay connected with those who really cared.

On a different level, their support also reminded me that

my peers still regarded me as a strong professional. The company had made a business decision, for better or worse. I needed to move on.

Not working gave me the freedom to focus on just me. I did what my doctor recommended and more. I designed my own therapy sessions, working on each issue that I identified. I am a researcher by nature, so I spent a great deal comparing different approaches, eventually trying Cowden, Buhner, Beyond Balance, Zhang and Byron White protocols. I joined many support groups to learn more about Lyme disease and the related issues.

From my research, I learned about and added far infrared sauna, PEMF, biomat, chi machine, Epson baths and a trampoline. It was slow going but I appreciated each new activity that I could do. Some days, in the beginning, the goals were small – stepping out into the backyard to feel the sunshine. That goal grew to taking long walks around the neighborhood. I would tackle tasks around the house, starting with just picking up things around the house until eventually, I was able to mow the lawn and do minor repairs. I rediscovered my local library. It became a place to read the paper, do my research, find fun topics to learn about or to rent movies or tv shows that I had always wanted to see but never had the time. I found free activities in the area which got me out of the house and engaging with others.

Eventually, I felt ready to go back to work. I was physically strong enough and ready to engage with the demands of others. I added networking, attending professional meetings and the usual job hunting tasks to my daily activities. I knew it would probably take a while for me to find the right job. It had been a while since I had been on the job market and I was insecure facing job hunting.

I found a woman at the local employment services office who helped me to be more confident in my job search. Together, we worked on my resume and practiced how to answer the hard questions about why I left my previous role. I was so fortunate that old friends who kept an eye out for opportunities. They kept my spirits up with lunches and messages, and forwarded along opportunities that they thought I might want to look at. I was lucky to find part-time contract work to ease into the workforce. It took a while but I found a job that I am happy with. The company is much more honest and understanding than my previous company.

My Lyme journey has been 6 years so far. It hasn't been a straight road. There were lots of twists and turns in the road. But I have to say that I am stronger for it.
In closing, I would like to share my lessons learned in case you are facing similar challenges:

- Be kind to yourself. You deserve it.
- Educate yourself about your health issues and actively participate in making decisions.
- Surround yourself with people who support you, both physically and emotionally.
- Understand that change is not always bad, especially if you take the time to assess each crossroad as an opportunity to grow.

Lyme Warrior
by Jennifer Heath

Before I was diagnosed with Lyme disease, I was a stay-at-home mom of three children, who are all grown. For fourteen years, I was a Top Leader, Recruiter, New Business Developer, and National Conference Trainer for Silpada Designs, a Direct Sales Company that is now out of business.

In March of 2013, I became deathly ill after a routine dental appointment. At the time, I didn't know the correlation between the dental appointment and my declining health. My illness baffled my team of doctors and specialists.

In August 2014, I was finally diagnosed with Lyme Disease, after going thru four surgeries and almost dying after the first. I was shocked to learn that after two weeks of antibiotics, and now bedridden, all of my doctors claimed that they do not treat Lyme Disease and the one doctor who would treat Lyme Disease had a three month waiting list.

I had no idea that my health was going to take a turn for the worse, before I would have to fight for my life to get better. I definitely wasn't expecting Lyme disease to make me relive the feelings of not feeling worthy or the sense of shame that I had suffered as a child due to being molested and abused. Yes, thanks to the 'Powers that be' not allowing Chronic Lyme Disease to exist, Lyme victims suffer from all kinds of abuse like: denied health care, or being socially ostracized, abandoned by their families and friends, spending their life savings on trying to get better, denied disability, and pretty much left for dead, like I was.

I didn't even know what Lyme disease was. All I knew was that after two weeks of antibiotics and now pronounced cured, I was now bedridden and left for dead by my doctors and specialist that had diagnosed me with other diseases prior to my Lyme diagnosis. Here are some of the diseases I was diagnosed with: chronic pain (fibromyalgia), calcified lymph nodes on my sternum, hypothyroid, synovial cyst, dense breast tissue, fibroid cystic breast disease, granulomas disease, edema, hypertension, bone spurs, spinal stenosis, degenerative disks, herniated disks, twisted vertebrae, tilted pelvis, uterine fibroids, ovarian cyst, shortness of breath, anemia, high estrogen levels, Adenomyosis, and medical menopause.

If you told me that my husband of 23 years, whom was very supportive of me up until my Lyme diagnosis, was going to believe the doctors that I was no longer sick with Lyme and forbid me to seek alternative treatments, I would have told you, 'No way!' If you were to tell me that some of my closest friends and family members were going to think I was just depressed and needed medication for my depression, I would have said, 'No way!'

Since only 2% of the medical community believes that Chronic Lyme Disease exists, I had no choice but to seek alternative medicine if I wanted to live. I don't believe I would be alive today without the direction and wisdom of my knowledgeable Naturopathic Doctor, Dr. Richard Easterling.

Thankfully, Dr. Easterling had moved to Tennessee 10

years prior to my diagnosis and was already knowledgeable about how to treat Lyme disease. He knew that I had to treat all the critters, a.k.a. parasites, viruses, bacteria, fungi, and Candida with holistic medicine. One can address all 5 of these at once, unlike one can do using synthetic drugs from Big Pharma, you just have to know how.

In my FREE Overcoming Lyme Disease Handbook, you can learn the secrets to what I did to heal my body of chronic pain and things that you can do from home to stay well. http://overcominglymedisease.com/%20free-handbook/

I continue to treat Lyme like Cancer. I am currently addressing a new cancer scare but I am not giving up nor backing down. In fact, I am fighting harder to stay well so I can start a nonprofit that will educate doctors on the true case definition of Lyme disease, which is relapsing fever aka Post-Sepsis or a B-CELL AIDS-like disease. I am also a dedicated Lyme Warrior advocate who wants to see the criminals responsible for the Lyme Crime mentioned in my book prosecuted for what is

being called, 'The Greatest Crime Against Humanity.'
If you want to stay informed and up to date on the latest
news about Lyme and health tips, download my free
handbook or register your name and email on my
website: http://www.overcominglymediseae.com

Jennifer Heath is the International Bestselling Author of,
'Overcoming Lyme Disease.' The book is called,
Overcoming Lyme Disease and not Overcame Lyme
Disease, because Lyme is a systemic disease like
cancer, which means that if you want to survive, you
need to treat it holistically.

https://overcominglymedisease.com/

Tough Diagnosis

By Laurie Penner

At the beginning of 2014, I noticed a severe mental decline. My job as a fiscal tech for Siskiyou County, California, involved contracts and spreadsheets, and I found myself suddenly unable to concentrate or follow everything. I'd scored very high on the fiscal testing for the job two years before, even at age fifty-nine. I had been diagnosed with fibromyalgia several years prior, so I was used to a certain amount of pain and fatigue, but suddenly losing mental capability was terrifying. My boss was very kind. I think he had decided it was my age that was the problem. But I knew it couldn't be that. I knew something was seriously wrong.

With a jury summons in hand — a job I knew I couldn't handle at the moment — I went through three doctors trying to get help. The first doctor told me to take pain meds and do my civil duty. I wasn't happy and made an appointment elsewhere. The next doctor found a low Vitamin B12 level and suggested I take that and come back in two months. He gave me a note to get off jury duty for a month. By this time, I had numbness in my left jaw and arm, heart palpitations, tingles and twitching on my skin, excessive sweating, low body temperature (which the nurse informed me was normal), and a multitude of other symptoms. I was hopeful about the B12, but even after my B12 level was much higher, I felt no better, except for less heartbeat issues.

The third doctor gave me an anti-depressant, a muscle relaxant and a prescription for physical therapy. She seemed to think I'd been sitting around too much and that's what caused the fatigue. She kept asking if I was getting any exercise. I wish! How could I explain that my lack of energy was not normal? I'd been very active before! My husband and I had just finished building a house over a period of six years, and I was still working on flooring and trim, and gardening every day when the debilitating fatigue hit. I'd even been hiking just a few months before and was hardly a couch potato! And why the anti-depressant? I refused it, since I was already on anti-anxiety medication that had worked for years.

Apparently, the fatigue droop made me look depressed.

I had grown emotionally dysfunctional. I thought it was from lack of answers. The muscle relaxant actually caused a deep depression! So much for that one. Then a co-worker suggested Lyme Disease. When I looked into it, I got excited about the symptoms but didn't think that could be it. I didn't remember being bit by a tick and I didn't have the famous bulls-eye rash. It wasn't until I discovered a large percentage of Lyme victims don't know they've been bit, due to the nymph tick being so tiny. Another large percentage don't get the rash. Could I possibly fit into both categories? I remembered pulling something bloody out of my left ear, the same side of my numbness. Could it have been a nymph tick?

Six months after I got so sick, my third physician gave me a round of Azithromycin, just in case there was a lingering infection. I didn't notice any improvement. But fortunately, I had read about how Lyme bacteria can hide in the body tissues, so I was not dissuaded from the Lyme possibility. I made an appointment with a Lyme Literate Naturopathic Doctor (LLMD) an hour away from me, in Oregon. My insurance wouldn't cover it and I would have to pay for everything out of pocket. I did this after much prayer, since my third doctor finally tested me for Lyme and got a negative report. Still, I persisted with the new appointment, because I'd heard a large percentage of Lyme tests show a false negative. All of the prior knowledge and information about Lyme that I had obtained helped tremendously, or I may have given up. I felt drawn to pursue the Lyme infection theory, no matter what, which I attribute to God's guidance. Three weeks later, the LLMD tested me again and it came out positive!

Wow. How many different ways could I beat the odds? That initial perseverance came in handy over the next few years as I followed natural protocols, mostly those of Stephen Buhner, for the Lyme and several co-infections my LLMD found. The mental decline made a quick turnaround at the beginning of treatment, thank God. Although I could tell the difference myself, a good indicator was in the word games I played with my sister. When I first got so sick, I had to make mostly three- or four-letter words, and I played at a medium challenge level with the computer as an opponent. It still beat me at that level. A year later, I started making a lot of "bingos"— seven-letter words or longer. Even on the expert level, I sometimes beat the computer. I was so relieved to get my brain back!

I could have been really upset with my local doctors, but I also had toxic mold in my body, with symptoms similar to Lyme Disease. Other infections like Babesia and Bartonella had also joined the bandwagon of hidden infections. So, even if the local doctors had found Lyme, I would doubtless have carried these other things inside me for some time. I'd also read that late-stage treatment of Lyme did not work well with the standard antibiotics that the local doctors would have used. So, even if they'd diagnosed me correctly, I wouldn't have gotten well.

The medical community doesn't usually test for toxic mold. One local doctor told me this. With all the fuss about toxic mold after flooding, you'd think they would. I discovered the mold had likely infected me in our leaky mobile home residence of eighteen years, probably due to my weakened immune system. Good thing we had built a house and moved out of there! I'd likely had the Bartonella over forty years, with symptoms I'd thought were mostly my own personality issues — like sudden rage and chronic anxiety, which dissipated with the natural treatment. The Babesia symptoms of chills, drenching night sweats, appetite issues, heart issues, and low blood pressure, had struck me the same time as the Lyme bacteria, so the Babesia bacteria probably arrived with the tick bite.

Three years after starting treatment for all of the above, my LLMD also found Chlamydia Pneumonia (CPN), a bacterium that can linger in the lungs and cause respiratory symptoms when the immune system goes down. I'd had a chronic cough for over twelve years that the doctors insisted was from allergies — including three ear, nose, and throat (ENT) specialists. I had tried every cough remedy recommended and never had any consistent relief. I coughed all day long, often out of control and embarrassing. Sometimes this cough was violent, causing a lot of misery and concern. It went away in about a year on the natural Buhner treatment for CPN.

My neural symptoms faded gradually over four years. The arthritis took several years to recover from, as well. My husband had to rub a special ointment that my LLMD made, down my neck and spine every night, so I could sleep better. After a while, I needed this less and less, until I didn't need it at all.

I still have the fatigue. But since I'm now sixty-five years old, and most definitely out of shape, I'm not sure anymore how this is still related to infection. Also, there could be yet another hidden infection that needs treatment. So, since I've done well in so many other ways, I just keep praying and trusting that God will guide me to complete wellness.

Battling various odd diseases over the years, Laurie has struggled with getting a correct diagnosis through standard medicine. She had written about her health issues, and the amazing near-death experiences of her husband, in a series of books called "Something's

Wrong." (New books, coming soon.) This series is intended to encourage both natural treatment and prayer, and to encourage others who suffer from hidden maladies or have a loved one in a health crisis.

https://www.amazon.com/Laurie-Penner/e/B00ITZ1L9C

ONE bite...just ONE

by Carole Kamerman

I worked hard all my life leading up to retirement. As so many others, I looked forward to retirement with much excitement. After all, I had put away a little retirement "nest egg" so that I could travel and see the things I had so anticipated upon retirement. It wasn't easy to save that money but I knew that the reward would be worth the sacrifice. I retired and then...I woke up one day with an insect bite on my right calf that developed a bullseye around it. It took forever to heal and the bullseye accompanied that bite the entire time. I went to the doctor 3 times and even suggested that it could possibly be a tick bite and I was worried about Lyme Disease. He stated, "We don't have Lyme Disease around here. It's just a spider bite." I knew very little about Lyme but friends had mentioned it enough times that I thought it was worth a mention. I was very concerned about the fact that the bite had this big round red ring around it.

Long story short...after this arrogant doctor denied that it could be Lyme and refused to treat me, misdiagnosed

70

me with MS and basically alluded to the fact that it was "all in my head," I found a doctor who tested, treated and supported me. She still does to this day as I went so long undiagnosed and untreated that I now have chronic Lyme. I still struggle with many symptoms, particularly neurological and cardiac issues. This is one LONG, difficult journey…at times very discouraging.

As my fellow retirees were traveling the world and heading to warmer climates during the winter months, I was shuttled back and forth to treatments and spent inordinate amounts of time bedridden…unable to attend social events with friends or even, at times, unable to walk out to my mailbox to get my mail. My "nest egg" was spent to pay for my treatments as insurance (still to this day) doesn't cover any of them. Depressing? Yes. But…I am GRATEFUL that I had that "nest egg" and am also glad that I have a few friends that understand what I cope with and are willing to stand by me. I have a family who understands how every day is a "crap shoot"…never knowing what each day brings. These people boost me up when I need it and encourage me. They celebrate my "good days" with me and we have fun! I no longer wake up each and take the day for granted. I have a "new normal" for now and if a cure for Lyme Disease is ever discovered, I will rejoice!! In the meantime, I have learned many lessons throughout this journey...some of them were tough to accept but I try not to think back on "what was" and look forward to each day as it comes. It makes no sense to try to compare my past to my present. I am becoming a brand new person who no longer takes her life for granted. It's the best I can do.

It's important to know that time is of the essence. If you suspect or know that you have been bitten by a tick make sure to pursue a diagnosis and treatment as soon as possible. The earlier a person gets treated, the more likely he or she will not suffer long term issues from Lyme Disease. If your doctor blows off the possibility, as mine did, go elsewhere. Don't let one doctor determine your fate.

One more important thing...ticks don't discriminate. You don't have to be an outdoorsy type person to be at risk. I am quite sure that the tick that bit me hitchhiked into my house on the fur of one of my dogs. I had found a few ticks questing in my house on the carpet, on my sofa…just about anywhere! I was always extremely careful when I was outdoors walking in the woods, working in the yard, attending outdoor concerts, etc. I knew that ticks could be a problem and had read about ways to minimize the likelihood of exposure to them. However, I did not realize that there were so many ticks in my community. There really was not much media coverage or hype in regard to issues about Lyme or ticks from our local television station or local newspaper.

The idea that Lyme could be a real threat for me seemed extremely unlikely but not impossible. And I really had no idea about chronic Lyme Disease. In fact, I didn't even know that it existed!!! My knowledge was basically this: If you get bitten by a tick get tested and then take some antibiotics and you would be cured…easy-peasy.

Things I wish I'd known: I wish I had known that if you didn't get treated fairly quickly that you could end up suffering the rest of your life…with chronic Lyme symptoms. In my case, neurological issues and cardiac issues remain with me yet today. It's so hard to think about the fact that if I had been treated with antibiotics when I went to the original doctor with that tick bite and bullseye I most likely would not be suffering yet today. I also wish I had an understanding that most Lyme tests are poorly designed and very unreliable. And finally, I wish I had known how important that bullseye around my tick bite was…it's a classic sign that I had been infected. I should have pursued treatment early on but I didn't know. I was uninformed.

Through the course of this disease I have lost: quality of life (once vibrant and active), friends (or those whom I thought were friends), ability to work or even volunteer, much of my retirement savings, security and confidence (as each day is unpredictable)…sometimes having to cancel plans or appointments due to symptom flares, and independence (having to depend on others when I am having an exceptionally difficult day.)

Through the course of this disease I have gained: a

new perspective on life, a new "normal," a circle of real friends who are there for me no matter what, opportunities to support others through this journey rather than wallow in self pity, the ability to say no when I need to, and the ability to bounce back and be grateful for any and all "good" days that come my way.

This is not an easy life. It is not what I expected. I struggle. I cry. But ultimately I thrive.

My advice to healthy people, young and old...enjoy every day. Don't wait until you retire to travel or try new things. Be adventurous. You never know when your life could change...by ONE tick bite...just ONE.

So Tiny, So Big

by Candice Mallicoat

The beginning of the year 2011 was joyfully filled with new changes and new life. My husband, our two children and I moved into a beautiful, large home and were expecting a new addition to our family. Six months after that baby was born, as we were enjoying our new home and neighborhood, I discovered a circular mark on my leg. It looked like a bullseye. A few days prior I had thought a clogged pore had created a blemish and I had squeezed it to release the pus. I thought this rash was rather odd for a blemish to result in a circular rash. I proceeded to a primary care physician who took a brief look at it and told me to "keep an eye on it" but it was probably just a bug bite. The next day I intuitively felt that there was more to the story. The rash was on my skin so I decided to see what a dermatologist would have to say. The doctor walked in, took one look at it and said, "That looks like Lyme disease." I asked him what Lyme disease was and he proceeded to tell me it was a tick borne illness. Oh dear, could that blemish actually have been a tick?! He didn't want to talk too much about it until he biopsied the rash. He seemed hesitant to believe that it was Lyme disease in Utah, after all I hadn't traveled anywhere out of state or even been camping.

In total naiveté I went home and waited for results. The doctor got back with me later that day which was rather quick I had thought, and delivered the news that my biopsy showed "indicative of Lyme." The blemish was not a blemish but a nymph sized tick apparently, so tiny I couldn't even tell it was a bug. I thought that it was not so bad; I'd take some meds and get over the infection. Yep, still quite naive. Then the doctor told me that he did not know where to send me for treatment and I was confused. He admitted that many doctors in our area would not take me seriously or treat me the way I really needed to be treated since they weren't very Lyme literate. That scared me. However, while I was waiting for test results, my husband had spoken to a co-worker whose wife had Lyme and was being treated successfully with a naturopath in our area. I told the dermatologist that I had someone I could see that was familiar with Lyme but he was a naturopath. I was encouraged to do whatever I could, as quickly as I could. That scared me too.

So the next few days were spent doing massive research. And I became even more scared. Lyme was not something I was going to just "take some meds for and get better" in a few weeks. I read about people with brain swelling, organ failure, dementia, nervous system issues, wheelchair bound, and psychotic symptoms and had no idea how Lyme was going to affect me. A week or two after diagnosis, my husband bless his heart, was telling me about more things he'd read about Lyme and I asked him to stop. I had read and learned a whole lot and the stress of what my life might be like was only going to make things worse. I had learned enough, had a treatment plan in place, and I wanted to put my head down and focus on walking through the fires of hell. Treatment started when I had a husband who worked 50 hours a week, a 4,500 square foot home to care for, a 6 month old, a 5 year old, and a 15 year old. I was a freelance copywriter with dreams to go to school and further my writing career. Yet, October 2011 changed everything. I was in so much pain during treatment that my body hurt and I was too weak to hold my baby. I would put her on a blanket, get on my hands and knees and drag her from room to room. I would grocery shop while trying not to vomit and I'd be so short of breath that it elicited odd looks from fellow shoppers. I could not tolerate the sounds of people talking, music, or TV. Every single joint in my body hurt, ached, and throbbed every single day and I was unable to continue work as a copywriter. A couple of times I even had neurological symptoms so bad that when someone was speaking to me it sounded like another language and I simply could not comprehend English. Awkward! My skin hurt so bad that my husband and I would have sex with me as fully dressed as possible to reduce the pain of him touching me. I had panic attacks multiple times a month and had trouble even making simple decisions on what to wear or how to do my hair; I'd be frozen and in tears from being unable to make decisions. Showering wiped me out for an hour, I'd be found curled up in front of infrared lights each evening when my husband came home because I was so chilled, and for weeks I'd wake up in the night feeling like my bones were on fire. Worst. Pain. Ever.

I was angry, scared, irritable, and realized the pain of chronic illness had taken the worst parts of my personality and made them even worse. My kids had the run of the house, I was often a momster, I was not active in their schooling as much as I wanted to be, and I could see they felt kind of abandoned. I saw the strain it put on my husband who tried so hard to be a rock of support every day and it broke my heart.

At some point after the first year I realized that this was going to be a longer journey than I thought. I felt that I had to have faith in healing or I would succumb to depression and possibility suicide. Even in my darkest hours I held onto a glimmer of a vision of health and vitality that I would someday reclaim. No matter how in despair I was, I couldn't shake that tiny bit of hope that I'd feel better and "normal" again.

Then one day I took a look in the mirror and realized I'd not showered for over a week, I had a ripe body odor cloud that followed me everywhere, and I didn't recognize who I was anymore. I had been so busy just getting through each damn day and nursing myself that I didn't even know what it was like to have hobbies or be a person any more. And to my sad reflection in the mirror I said, "ENOUGH! I will not let this illness run and ruin more of my life than it has to."

That changed everything! I was now in a place of acceptance, rather than resentment or resistance, to the illness I experienced. I practiced deep self-love and got serious with daily treatment and detox protocols. I wrote in a gratitude journal, attended spiritual and personal growth workshops, I traveled with my family, and sang karaoke. I went to costume parties and did crafts. And you want to know what? I did all of that in the middle of treatment. I did it even when I was nauseated, headachy, woozy, forgetful, fatigued, weak, short of breath, and more. I often experienced 40 symptoms per day but I would go out and do all of this anyway.

I started to sense the woman behind the illness. She started to fight and thrive. She continued to seek answers for health and try new things, and she started to shift the healing energy in abundance ways.

Over the course of 2 years we used antibiotics, oregano

oil, cat's claw, banderol, strong homeopathic remedies, liposomal vitamin C, chelation therapy, UV IV's, and dozens upon dozens of herbal supplements to support my body. Then finally around the two and a half year mark my test results and symptoms showed Lyme was gone, or in remission at the very least. From Lyme infection in 2011 to the point that I felt the healthiest and most whole took about seven years. During that time I dealt with babesia, bartonella, numerous other Lyme co-infections, staph infections, intestinal parasites, mold illness, discoid lupus, cytomegalovirus, Epstein Barr virus, malnourishment, leaky gut, and more.

It was not easy, by any stretch of the imagination, but through it all I never expected to receive so many blessings from the experience or heal myself so well. It's been a journey I was supposed to take so that I can now teach others how to awaken their inner healing abilities and higher selves. From my mess came my message that I share from my business, Embody Wellness Coaching where we take a mind, body, spirit approach to self-healing that is effective and intuitive. I appreciate spreading awareness about this rotten disease so people grasp the importance of tick prevention and learn about tick borne illness. I also hope to be of inspiration to others out there who have yet to heal. The body's capacity to overcome serious trials is amazing. The journey might not be short but a hefty dose of patience, peppered with faith and determination, can bring miracles.

Lyme Diary

by Cassidy Colbert

Growing up in Maryland, Lyme disease was prevalent, but I never truly understood this horrible disease, until I got it myself.

In May of 2012, when I was fourteen, I got a headache that would not go away. I started sleeping all the time, and the pain soon spread to every inch of my body. My mom took me to a neurologist, who was no help. He ordered a brain MRI, which didn't show anything, so he decided I must need anti-depressants to help me sleep. Then we went to an orthopedist, who did an x-ray of my head and told me that I had severe arthritis in my neck. All I could think was "how do I, a healthy fourteen year old, get arthritis?" Luckily, my mother thought the same thing.

So, we continued going to many other doctors and specialists, trying to find answers. I was diagnosed with chronic fatigue syndrome, chronic tension headaches, Ankylosing Spondylitis, and finally, Fibromyalgia.

However, I never seemed to fit completely into any of these diagnoses. That is when Lyme disease came into the picture.

We had known a few people who had Lyme disease, but we never knew much about it. Luckily, a close family friend, who happened to be an avid adventurer and ER doctor, told us about Chronic Lyme Disease. She helped us find a Lyme Literate doctor, and my true Lyme journey began.

I will admit that when I got diagnosed with Lyme, I was relieved. I thought "Oh Lyme disease? That is easy! They can clear this up very quickly and I will be good as new!" I thought. I was very, very wrong.

At my very first appointment, I was taken aback. My doctor was talking about a protocol going months into the future, a bill way higher than my usual $20 co-pay, and I had the most vials of blood taken (at the time) that I had ever seen. This is when it first hit me how real Lyme disease really is.

Over the next few months, things started getting worse. My brain function started deteriorating, and my stomach issues began. It was then that we decided to try the holistic route. However, after a few months and over $2,000, I saw no improvement, so we started from ground zero.

I ended up finding a new Lyme literate doctor, who I saw for two years. With this doctor, we found out that I had the co-infections Babesia, Bartonella, and Mycoplasma. We also discovered that I have a gene mutation, MTHFR, which makes it harder for me to heal. We treated with oral antibiotics for a long time, but my stomach got worse, which led us to getting my first PICC, peripherally inserted central catheter, line.

After a month with the PICC, I saw the most improvement I had ever seen-I went from being 30% recovered to about 80% recovered. This improvement kept up for the next 8 months that I had the PICC. In fact, things were going so well that I was headed off to college, and basically in remission when the PICC came out. However, the good feelings were short lived, as I was exposed to mold, and I relapsed hard about three weeks into school. It got so bad that I could not read anymore, and started getting partial paralysis. So, I was forced to leave school.

When I came home, I got my second PICC line. I saw improvement with this one, but it took longer than the first PICC. I had this PICC for 9 months, but unfortunately, I got a blood clot in my left lung, and had to have it removed. After this, we tried to treat with oral antibiotics, and I was functioning alright, but not 100%. It got to the point that I just needed a break from treatment to try and rebuild my body, so I stopped treatment last April.

I actually had been doing all right, going to school and working part-time. However, this past fall, I started deteriorating again. So we have started treatment back up, and I am slowly getting better. I am at the point mentally, where I am ready to do anything to feel well again including not eating gluten, dairy, sugar, or grains. Getting better is a full-time job. I have to calculate when to take medicines, what I can, and cannot eat, and what

I am able to. It is a lot for a person, and while I try to stay positive, the depression finds me every now and then.

The first time I sunk into depression with Lyme, was a year after my first symptoms began, in May of 2013. I do not think anyone really ever knew how bad it truly got, but let's just say it was dark and scary, and I never want to get back there. One day when I was noticeably depressed, my sister suggested I start a blog to share my story. At first, I was hesitant. "Do I really want people knowing my business?" "What if no one reads it?" "Is this stupid?" These were all questions I asked myself. Finally, I decided to do it.

In May of 2013, I started Thelymediary.wordpress.com, and my life changed for the better. I quickly learned that I was not alone in my struggles. I started getting messages from other lymies, lending support and their own stories. I found some support groups on Facebook and joined them. However, I quickly realized that most of the people in these groups were adults who did not have the same problems that I did. Sure we all had pain and tremors, but while they were worrying about taking care of their kids, I was worried about getting to school to see my friends.

It was then that I decided to create my Teens with Lyme Facebook page. I like to think that this page, and my blog, saved my life. It was through these avenues that I found my Lymie family. Even though I have never met these people in real life, I am closer to them than anyone else. I share my deepest secrets, weirdest symptoms, and pain with them. The group started off slowly, but suddenly, I was getting 10-15 new member requests a day. Today, there are over 400 members in my group, from all over the world. It amazes me how much love there is in the lymie community. I would do anything for these people, and I know they feel the same way about me.

It was also through the group, and my blog, that I got more involved in the advocacy side of Lyme disease. We attended May Day rallies, walked in the Loudon Lyme walk, and post about Lyme disease everywhere! My saying is "Awareness is Key," and I believe that with all my heart. We will never get the coverage, care, and recognition we deserve if no one knows what we are going through. That is why I share my story. That is why I talk about the bad stuff. It may be gross, and sad, but that is what Lyme disease is.

So when I was asked, in the spring of 2016, to testify in front of the Maryland State House and Senate on a new Lyme disease bill, I was thrilled. At this point, I had been sick for 4 years, had dropped out of college, and got my second PICC line, so passion for change was not lacking. I got up there and told my story, along with a few other sufferers, and a few weeks later, the bill passed. This bill requires that doctors inform people that if their blood test comes back negative for Lyme, they could still have it. This may seem like a little thing, but for the Lyme community, it was monumental.

If I had known about the poor testing when I first started showing symptoms, my Lyme could have been caught sooner, and in turn, I could have potentially gotten better sooner. So if this bill helps just one person get a diagnosis, and feel better, I will be pleased.

This is why I was ecstatic to be asked to testify again, this past February, on a new Lyme bill. This bill would require the insurance companies to cover Lyme disease treatment for as long as the doctor deems necessary-which would be great for me since we owe over $60,000 for my PUCC. Although we still do not know the outcome of this bill yet, our stories were heard and that is all that matters.

I have seen people lose their homes, lose their chance at an education, lose friends, and most importantly, lose their lives from this disease. On the other hand, I have seen people recover from this disease, and live normal, successful lives.

People underestimate lymies. Just because we are chronically sick does not mean we are weak. In fact, it means just the opposite. We are out here fighting for the most important thing in the world-our lives. While the journey may be long, and awfully bumpy, and at some points seems never ending, I have hope that one day there will be an end. One day, I will reach remission, because, if one person can get there, then we all can.

Cassidy Colbert writes a blog called "Lyme Diary" at https://thelymediary.wordpress.com/ and a vlog on youtube called Lyssa & Lyme: https://www.youtube.com/channel/UC5e5LuWxrkLjVuY1L8aPAvg

Just a Tick

by Niki Slovacek

September 2002

Helping close the pool at my parents' house I reached up to pull my hair back in a pony tail, barley 8 weeks pregnant. I felt a hard "scab" behind my ear, I called for my dad to see what it was.

"Just a tick" he said, but I called my OB-GYN to get advice. They insisted I had to come in and get it removed right away. I drove the 30 minutes and they pulled it off. I had a red welt but they insisted I Was fine; they showed me "textbook" pictures for a bullseye rash and toll me I just had a reaction like I would if I had a mosquito bite. I believed them.

During the pregnancy with Chase I was hospitalized for horrible dizzy spells, massive migraines, joint pain etc., at 24 weeks I went into preterm labor. Contractions slowed down but never totally stopped. I delivered Chase on April 4th 2003, he was blue in color, couldn't cry and had difficulty breathing. The Drs at the hospital wouldn't listen so we went home.

On day three of Chases life we took him to a pediatrician that took me seriously over the phone. He saw Chase and ran tests immediately, he had a serious infection and no idea where it came from. We headed to a children's hospital that was expecting us. After many, many tests they told us that chase had infections everywhere in his body. Eyes, lungs, mucus, urine etc. loaded with infection. They looked for the cause, none was to be found. They were befuddled and stopped looking. Chase had two IV's in him, one with constant IV antibiotics of two sorts, the other for meds and fluids. We sat there for almost three weeks with no answers. Eventually they let us go without answers, we let it go. Life went on.

July 2006 I gave birth to my daughter Gabi, no complications or issues during pregnancy.

Soon after birth Gabi had constant problems with her eyes. She screamed all night long, I kept her mattress propped up and sought help. The ENT said there was lots of pressure behind her ears but no infection. Month after month we found no cause. At a year old she had tubes put in her eyes. Her doctor said that when she put the tubes in there was a rush of pressure that came out but no fluid. The ear pain stopped but within three month she would start having seizures that were unexplained. They struggled to find a cause and insisted she would grow out of them. She was then diagnosed with juvenile RA and I was told to keep an eye on it as she got older. Motrin was need now for pain and possible other meds as she aged. I was frustrated and stressed. One doctor after another and no known cause. We were ignored and pushed aside. We were told over and over to treat the symptoms.

In 2011 I was pregnant with Tatijana, the pregnancy was hell. MY joint pain was incredible. I was in the shower for 60-90 minutes at a time begging God for relief. Doctors blew me off and said it was normal. We knew better. I couldn't function, my head pounded constantly and I nerve pain started to rear its ugly head.

In July gave birth to a 6 week premature little girl delivered by C-section. She was tiny and quite and took forever to grow. She wore preemie clothes for 6 weeks and newborn for 3 more months, all while being breastfed.

By December of 2011 my neck and head felt like it was constantly on fire and the pain was horrifying. It felt as if I need to remove my spine, opening a space for fluid to no longer be trapped in a space in needed to explode. We husband had me to specialist all over the tri-state area. MRI's, CAT scans, blood work and other tests were ran and no known cause was found. I was sick of hearing that, I left the specialists office crying. "Find it" I thought, but no one would. No one wanted to look for the "zebra", all they wanted was to diagnose an easy patient and collect a check.

By 2012 Gabi had contact anxiety attacks that kept her from playing, school and almost any public place. The sensitivity to light was so bad we ate with the dining room lights dimmed. Her constant tummy troubles, early puberty and muscle and joint pain were under control. I took her to the doctor for a pain injection and they gave her a steroid shot. Her pain was off the charts within 45 minutes and we were in the ER. They started an IV and made her comfortable. NO answers. I sat there and googled "worse pain after steroids" and Lyme Disease popped up immediately. Excited I started soaking up everything I could. I looked into symptoms and causes in the attempt to see if that was what was afflicting her. After three weeks of talking to her doctor we sent both of our blood work out to a specialty company, it would take four weeks to get the results. We waited with baited breath.

The results came in and we had answers. Both of us were so excited to know we could fight this, until we found out that insurance rarely covers treatments and getting into a LLMD could take up to six months. We didn't care, we had answers.

While there is no current cure or solid treatment plan for Lyme, we have spent thousands traveling to doctors, buying supplements and paying for traditional medication. Chase was never tested by sending in blood samples but suffers the same joint pain (not nearly as bad) and anxiety that comes and goes with no outlying cause.

We fight on.

My Lyme Journey

By John Coughlin

I am sharing this because I want all my friends to know my Journey and not trying to jinx myself into relapse or looking for attention etc. Just want to show how much I have gone through to get to where I am now.

Heart palps including fluttering and pounding and skipping. (haven't had the fluttering and pounding in years now, but think I still have some damage from having Lyme so long and all the treatments etc.) drank a lot grape juice and berry juices to keep my heart strong..

Skin problems, bumps in my scalp, skin rashes showing up in different parts of body, some raised and some blotchy and some like bartonella-like scratches .. (bumps in my scalp would scab up and peel off in a couple of weeks) Haven't had this in about three years now it's been good to go.

Fatigue problems.. in the onset the fatigue on a scale of 1 to 10 was a 10 plus and continued as a 7 or 8 most of the time (extreme fatigue issues) I still have fatigue issues but nothing like the onset in 99 things are much more manageable now.

Itchy skin, buggy feeling like bugs crawling in my skin.. I get this once in a blue moon now but nothing like when I was on treatments and felt like scratching my skin off, it was so annoying.. muscle spasms, cramps in hands and legs and shooting pains up my legs, muscle twitching, shooting pains up and down my legs, restless leg at night when laying down. I still have problems with vibrations in legs when I stand too much or take on too much activity in a day.

Muscle twitching still comes and goes but not nearly as often as before.. Sometimes just opening a jar would make my hand cramp up with unbelievable pain..stiffness in my legs in the morning would limp around the house, felt like my legs were locking up.. Much, much better now do not have this in the morning anymore.. Thank God..buzzing and shaking in my legs like my legs were plugged into an electric socket.. Can happen any time of the day or night mostly from over activity I think, but not really sure about that..Noise and Light sensitivity mostly on the onset and subsided a lot after combo abx treatments. Could not even look at the computer screen is bothered my eyes, but pretty much all gone now but I wouldn't go looking into the Sun lol even a normal person wouldn't do that.. Double vision, would last about 10 to twenty minutes and then my eyes would turn to normal.. Got much better during and after treatments.. (dark sunglasses helped a lot) haven't had double vision now since 06 and i hope to God it never comes back.

Dizzy and foggy was very severe in the onset of the disease, carried all the way through at different levels until 3 years of combo treatments helped bring them to a very low level now almost normal now.. that outer space feeling is a thing of the past, hoping it stays that way.

Palsy like symptoms in left side of my face and numbness and tightening of face too.. Still have lingering symptoms of this that come and go only for short periods of time.. very limited range of motion in my right shoulder could not throw anything over hand with it just underhand.. Now I can throw over hand but not the same range of motion before Lyme.

Chest problems, including a wheezing, air hunger .. wheezing lasted for three months before it finally subsided .. (really felt like i was dying with this symptom) thank God it's all gone now and hope it never comes back again. Unexplained cough.. I still get this on occasion but nothing as often and severe as it was in the beginning of the illness.. Standing for long periods. Couldn't stand for too long, usually about 20 minutes max before i would get weary and need to sit down or lay down for a while.. Joint pain.. I didn't get any joint pain until about two years into it.. It was about six years from onset of first symptoms that my legs started to lock up and get stiff in the morning.

Memory problems.. In the onset first year was really bad.. could not remember close friends names that i should know like cream cheese.. still have trouble spelling simple words sometimes, it's like brain freeze maybe from brain damage not sure though..

Problems sleeping has been an issue waking up 3 o'clock in the morning, it's been like clockwork for quite a while .. now it's hit or miss some nights good and once in a while I still wake up early hours in the morning.. Sore throat would come and go at random, especially in the onset of illness and then would be off and on from there.. Now I don't have this problem for quite a good while now and hoping it stays that way, no jinx..

Light headed and brain fog was a big problem, was afraid to leave the house and go anywhere by myself.. felt like I was in outer space or space cadet or something.. felt like I was fainting all the time or going to faint, but now it's mostly gone and nothing like it was in the onset of illness. Severe dizzy was a big problem, if turn too fast the wrong way I could be on the floor in seconds with the room spinning round and round.. Sometimes the spinning would not stop and I ended up in the ER a few times, only to have the doc yell at me and tell me I didn't have Lyme when I did.. Now thank God the spinning has not happened in about 4 years but sometimes I feel like it could come back, very scary indeed, one of the worst Lyme symptoms in my opinion.

Shortness of breath and air hunger was a problem, but not as severe as some others on the net that got this way more severe than I.

Swollen Lymph nodes was a problem in the onset and one clinical doctor was sure it was from Lyme even though I had a ton of Lyme tests and doctors telling me I had Chronic Fatigue Syndrome, etc.. He was the only doctor that thought of lifting my arm and checking under my arm pits all the other docs were clueless he called them Nurses (lol). Rashes in the onset were very large and raised and troubling, very itchy and would stay up all night scratching and drawing blood at times, felt like I was in hell for sure. Then later on I had scratch like rashes showing up, especially after a hot shower would bring them out..

Concentrations issues was a big problem in the onset and through the beginning years of this whacky disease, there were times i could not concentrate for a minute on anything. Social services lady sent me to boces to learn about computers tech and I only lasted about 10 minutes in the classroom and had to get up and leave.. these people were clueless to late stage Lyme and what it does to people.

Balance issues was a big problem, had to watch myself on a ladder or doing things that require good balance.. fell off a ladder once and it took 3 months for my leg to heal. VA lady made me walk a straight line, when i just told her I have this problem and i fell over and almost hurt myself.. they just don't believe us or get it do they? very sad indeed being a Lymie.. White patches on my feet and legs like dried skin or something.. still have this issue but it really doesn't bother me much or itch etc. but they are still visible white dots on my feet and legs..

My Treatments: In '99 I had one clinical doc that was sure I had Lyme disease and I was doing Amoxicillin with probenecid 3000 mgs daily. I did that on and off for three years, a year on and then a year off etc. after a while I realized when I stopped the treatments it got worse, felt better while on the treatments. In '06 I got so bad I could hardly walk with severe dizzy attacks and double vision, it was then I realized that if I didn't do something fast I was going to be an invalid soon..

It was in '07 that I found a LLMD and had a PCR and Spect scan proving Lyme and Lyme damage to my brain. Took me two hospitals before I found one that knew what a spect scan was and had the equipment to do it.. Once my diagnosis I was taking doxy for about six months and wasn't getting much better.. I asked my LLMD if I could try a combo because some I knew were doing ceftin and biaxin at the time combination therapy oral antibiotics.

I was lucky to have two doctors one which was my primary and my Lyme Literate working together to help me get better. I figured if I didn't do or try something what would be the outcome then, wheelchair? Suicide? I just didn't want to live like this anymore so I decided for myself to go down fighting and treat the disease. I know everybody is different so I hope this helps a little that you would find your own protocol that would help you heal..

In between treatments especially when my heart was pounding and skipping I would take a drug holiday when I felt it was really necessary and would do some natural stuff, like oil of oregano drops under tongue.. Olive leaf extract and magnesium for twitching and spasms..

Helpful hints…

One of the biggest things that helped me get better is the wealth of information I found on the net, especially Dr. Burrascanos Lyme guidelines was big help.. www.lymenet.org/BurrGuide200810.pdf

Lyme symptom charts. http://lyme-symptoms.com/LymeCoinfectionChart.html

Late Stage patient information www.angelfire.com/me2/StarShar/Herx1.html

Having a LLMD (Lyme Literate MD) that is willing to work with you and try different things, mine was willing to switch things up when doxycycline wasn't working. Trying to find the right protocol for you and your situation is very important, LLMD's they have a lot of experience with this very often complicated disease. My Literate was also very good at reinforcing the idea that Chronic Lyme is a real disease and I have a big task ahead of me, she never said I would be completely cured but only said as time goes on I could get better from the Lyme, then we can go from there after the Lyme is treated and under control.

Dr. Alan MacDonald says that Lyme is hard to diagnose, treat and is capable of relapse, so having someone that has the right background dealing with Lyme patients all day long is your best bet in my opinion.. Unless you catch and treat the Lyme from day one with some antibiotics for at least 3 to 6 weeks you may end up Chronic, getting treating early in the game is so important but because docs are not properly trained or want to use antibiotics needlessly, they very often spin the wheel of fortune or misfortune with your life. If they guess right you will be ok and tick will be a dud but if they are wrong you could end up sick for the rest of your life, just ask the thousands of us online support groups who are now Chronic. Dr. Alan's work proves that ticks can have more than just Bb but also many other pathogens up to a dozen co infections have been found in ticks, and now a new virus in NY and Kansas.

A Dame Called Bartonella

By: Sam Bugala

I imagined the seasoned surgeon whistling to himself at the end of his shift, twirling the keys to his expensive new convertible around his manicured finger. He'd have a date set up, already showered with the scent of Old Spice replacing the sharp bite of antibacterial soap he'd doused both arms with. Rounding the corner to the parking garage the tune would catch in his throat, the keys crash to the concrete, when his lovely new lightning yellow Chevrolet had an Asian impaled through the canopy and splattered across the Corinthian leather, eyes still staring him down in manic glee. This thought brought a macabre grin to my face as I stood on the edge of a parking garage balcony outside a hospital. Horribly depressed, dreadfully confused, and finding joy in how my death would end with a bang like none other.

A good noir story needs a good noir dame, one shrouded in mystery and a name that could be a cross between a stripper or a princess. Her name was Bartonella, a little vixen that tongue rapes the brain and whispers sweet nothings to those dark place, she gave me sorrow and toyed with my mind with the wanton abandon of an overdose of happy pills.

But before I knew my vixens name, I enjoyed a plethora of emails and texts from other perspective "catfish". Their names were Bipolar (fun but emotional), Aspergers (standoffish but intelligent) and Schizophrenia (one kiss and your hooked for life). It wasn't until a suggestion from a Ms. Vickie, shed light on the true culprit. By this time the smell of hospital stench hung heavy in my hair and the chalky taste of every psychotropics lingered in my mouth like cigarette ash. Putting a name to the disease was like a parlor room scene where the detective names the killer. There was surprise, confusion, and the relief that the culprit wouldn't get away. But my dearest Bartonella remains quick on her feet and still sleeps peacefully in my skull, occasionally gnawing at my corpus collosum. She waxes and wanes in prevalence, some days feel like the weight of my skull will snap my spine, others I feel considerably better. But this was a story about struggle, hope, and the promises of tomorrows. Noir films usually don't follow that narrative, and neither does that dame Bartonella.

You want the story? Ink hasn't dried and plenty can happen with the well so close to the page, I spend my days writing about mysteries and adventures when I've yet to solve the mystery whether Bartonella was the Bipolar, Aspergers, and Schizophrenia or whether one will be left behind when she leaves. The road ahead is darker than a politicians soul, and colder than their hearts. Sometimes it takes the fires of words and dark humor to lift my spirits, other days the still steady doses of psychotropics. In the end, I think I'm asking too much when I ask for hope and give nothing in return. The imaginary man who fell from that parking garage made manic demands for hope that were never met. The man who took the elevator to ground level took a different approach, in his hands he held out optimism and the trade for hope was made. It's not the end most people want, but when I wade through the darkness while my vixen giggles and clacks her teeth, I hold out for the hope that she'll leave in the dead of night like the unfaithful succubus she is, and I'll wake out of my world of shadows. Maybe this hope will light the way.

The Fall

By George Popovici

My odyssey began in October 2005 when I started to feel pains in my groin and legs. I quickly made an appointment with my local primary care doctor, who happened to be a social friend of mine. I spoke to this man, who I called "Doc," with confidence about my difficulties—after all, throughout my entire life I had been in command of any and all crises. My belief that I was in command of life came from my experience as an emergency medical technician, a firefighter in my early years, and later in my current career as a safety engineer. (Safety Engineers solve all types of complex and technical problems). As with all engineers, we are trained to believe that there is a logical solution for every problem: A+B=C and so I thought we would easily find a solution to my medical issue as well.

Like most healthy Americans, I did not spend much time in doctors' offices or medical facilities. As a matter of fact, I avoided them like the plague. The notion of wasting any more of my precious life having an annual physical and hanging around a germ-infested waiting room with folks who were ill was completely repulsive to me. I felt I was far too important to my family and to those who I served in my work and in the community. When I first became ill, I was taken aback. "I am George Popovici," I told myself, "and this can't be happening to me."

Doc ran the usual blood tests, and based on my symptoms, he deduced that I had a prostate infection known as prostatitis. He prescribed a one-month course of heavy-duty antibiotics, which is the standard course of treatment for a malady of this nature. By Thanksgiving, a month later, I was very weak. Mind you, I was a 5'9" 145-pound granola-eating kayaker. I could outpace most men my age, and run with the best of them. I played with my kids, and enjoyed outrunning them whenever possible. As a matter of fact, I was "the Dad that could." I deep-sea fished, swam, downhill-skied, hiked, white-water rafted, hunted, and exercised regularly with weights and bike-riding. But I was barely able to stand while attending a charity auction in early December, and in fact, I had to sit through the entire event.

I had confidence in Doc, but knew deep down after the third clinical visit and associated laboratory tests that whatever was happening to me was highly unusual and very abnormal. Having been a healthy person all of my life, I knew my body, and what felt right and wrong. This was definitely wrong. I knew I should be starting to improve at this point, but the weakness and pain persisted. As a matter of fact, the pain had started to turn into a burning sensation in my thighs.

For the first time in my life, I began to doubt. Could the weakness have been a reaction to the antibiotics? Did I do more damage by taking the "big gun" pharmacological prescription? Why should I ask myself such questions? After all, I had faith in the medical community, and had no reason to question or doubt any medical professional. As an educated engineer, I understood the scientific advances made in medical science, knew many doctors socially, and listened to them speak of the new research or treatment regimens appearing for the benefit of their patients. Surely, Doc could find the underlying cause of my problem and order the proper treatment so I could get back to my very busy life.

Christmas was almost upon us, and we had to get the house ready for the kids. My firstborn son Nicholas was 14 at the time, my daughter Alexandra was 12, and little Gregory was 10. We were right in the thick of social events surrounding the holidays and planning winter activities.

On my fourth office visit, just before Christmas 2005, Doc told me he really did not have a clear clinical picture as to what was happening to me. I started to lose the "fuzzy feeling" I had about him as my situation worsened. My joints had started to ache excruciatingly every time I moved. Thankfully, my work is primarily in an office setting, so I was able to make my normal 75-minute commute and sit at my desk for most of the day. Walking to and from my car was a challenge, as I huffed and puffed. I had to carry my laptop computer and other critical safety data with me every day in case I was called on in the off hours of my job.

Doc finally sent me to a local hospital to test for Lyme disease, and simultaneously referred me to a rheumatologist friend of his in a neighboring community, Dr. Marcy, who he felt would have more in-depth specific training in obscure diseases. Sadly, I was told it would take me three months to see Dr. Marcy.

For those of you not familiar with Lyme disease, it is a bacterial infection in which spirochetes bore into the muscle tissue causing tremendous joint pain, neurological problems, and weakness. If left untreated, it can be fatal. Three months into the illness, my tests for the disease came back negative. What many doctors do not know about this insidious disease is that the standard testing is not conclusive at all times. Depending on the stage of the disease, it may show as negative on various tests.

Over the holidays, I spoke with family and friends as well as other physicians I was acquainted with. All of them urged me "not to fool around" and to get to a Boston Hospital. After all, Boston is a major city, with the oldest university in the nation. Extending my care to a city hospital was an idea that did not appeal to me, because I was trying to conceal my illness at this point. It was shameful to me for a host of reasons. The New Year was on the horizon, and I had big projects planned at work. My boss at the time was a good-hearted man; however, he was trained in the US Army and retired as a full Colonel. Although he did not say it, I knew he wanted me to "adapt and overcome" by keeping a stiff upper lip and bearing it out....and believe me I felt the same way! My symptoms had reached a point where I finally had a sit-down with him, and told him I had a health issue but that I expected to rapidly resolve it. He seemed to support this notion, and released me for a few hours over the next few weeks so I could get to the bottom of my illness.

"Ok," I thought, "now that I have a plan, who do I see? Where do I go?" There are many hospitals in Boston. Right then and there, I knew that I would have to advocate for myself. If you have not ever been in that space, it can be daunting, frustrating, lonely, and downright scary.

While I was at work, I confided in my friend Margaret Nunes. Mary is a young, successful, vibrant director in our corporate relations group at my company. Margaret is amazing in her outlook and spirit. She always hugs me when we meet, and generally has a smile on her face.

The way I became acquainted with Margaret was unusual, to say the least. I was walking the floor of a safety conference trade show in 2004 in Orlando. I started a conversation with a vendor who sold Automatic Electronic Defibrillators (AED's). When the vendor asked where I worked and I told him, he replied, "I am Margaret Nunes brother." After listening to his sales pitch, I emailed Margaret to introduce myself and tell her of my chance meeting. Little did I know that she would become a lifeline angel for me one year later.

I have come to understand that there are angels all around us all the time. We don't often recognize them because we are too caught up in our daily routine, or brush their messages off as coincidence. I am firmly convinced that Margaret's brother led me to her for a reason. This was my introduction to the angels who circled me and guided me as I fell further into ill health.

Now, before you think I have had one too many pharmacological injections, I will tell you that I was as skeptical as anyone at this point in my life. I am an engineer. I lived squarely in the linear, physical world, and have always reverted to the simple formula of A+B=C. It is incredible to me that these kinds of "coincidences" keep presenting themselves in my life.

Margaret has been diagnosed with rheumatoid arthritis. RA (as it is known) is a debilitating inflammatory disease that primarily affects the joints and other organs of the body. Margaret was being seen by a doctor whom she raved about, and she believed he could shed light on my advancing condition. His name was Dr. Richards , and he practiced at major Boston hospital. This medical facility is considered by many to be the premier medical facility in the nation. Margaret gave me Dr. Richards' name, and she also called her contact who was able to arrange a speedy appointment for this doctor who was in great demand.

By this point, I was falling into disbelief that my health could fail, and that I would become this ill this quickly without any answers. I was used to getting answers to my questions fairly quickly. My symptoms had progressed at this point—I was so weak I could barely walk; I had started to develop visual difficulties; my skin was getting mysteriously darker; and I noticed flashing lights when I closed my eyes.

I intentionally minimized my situation to my wife, because she was the commander of our home for day-to-day operations, and I felt that having her worry would only make matters worse at home. I had my appointment set for January 15th, 2006. The worry and wait had really taken its toll. Thankfully, the holidays were behind us, allowing me to focus on getting to the cause of my failing health.

Dr. Richards was an elderly but well-respected doctor. He listened patiently to me as I explained the expanding constellation of symptoms. I think he was truly receptive until I broke down emotionally. I started to weep like a child. He was polite and kind, but suspected that my illness was more of a psychological type than an organic variety. The pressure to find an answer and get back to normal business had taken its toll, right there in his Boston exam room.

Dr. Richards assured me that he would be back to me within a week. When the week had come and gone, I called. As with many practices, the nurse relays the laboratory findings to the patient, especially if the doctor has a busy practice or does not want to deal with the patient. In my case, I suspected the latter. At that time, the only abnormal labs were elevated protein in my blood and a higher-than-normal C Reactive Protein (CRP), which is a marker of inflammation. When I questioned the nurse, she felt it was not a matter of concern per the doctor's note, and said that he would not need to see me again. In effect, a dismissal. Conversely, when I called my local doc to get a second opinion, he indicated that these were significant findings. "Oh, great," I thought, "now what do I do?" This was my first encounter with a major medical facility, and I found it sadly lacking. I felt rejected and perplexed. A feeling that would repeat itself for years to come.

~ from Chapter 1 of George's book, *Angels Walking with Us*

---

for more information and Lyme Disease related resources click on:

www.angelswalkingwithus.net

Beyond Exhausted

by Carleen Eve Fischer Hoffman

For the past 16 years I've been dealing with fatigue. I don't mean the kind where you take a little nap and then feel better. I'm talking about down and out, drag your ass, unsafe to even drive kind of fatigue; the kind where some days you don't dare get in a car because you could endanger yourself and others. I was falling asleep at work and at class.

I've been to many doctors, done test after test with no results. I consulted with my primary care physician who kept testing me each year for the same things, including Lyme Disease. The tests always came back negative. I consulted with my OBGYN. I saw a pulmonary doctor (who was very handsome by the way). Eventually, I went back to my primary care physician and insisted that he do something else to help me. He suggested I have a sleep study done. I think he did this just to humor me.

I purchased a pair of classy pajamas with the letter "C"

on the pocket to mark the occasion. My husband drove me to the lab, where I was to stay overnight and sleep in front of a man I never met with all kinds of electrodes attached to my head and body. The test was unnerving. During the middle of the night I thought about asking the monitor man if he could bring me a snack just to see if he was actually awake. I only slept for two hours. When the morning came, monitor man decided I needed to stay an extra four hours for additional tests. I remember leaving the facility with all kinds of goop in my knotted hair and left with only an hour to get back to the house, shower, and be awake for the next five hours for a fancy event my husband and I had to attend. I made it through the event (my hair looked great!), and the sleep study came back with nothing useful.

The sleep doctor suggested I see his sleep shrink to discuss sleep habits. It was a disaster. At every appointment, as soon as I sat down, the sleep shrink would ask me if I paid my bill for the previous visit before proceeding with the appointment. I decided that if all he cared about was whether or not I paid my bill I didn't care to see him anymore!

A few years went by and I continued to deal with the frustration of the fatigue. Some days I would be ok, other days I would have to nap. I still tried to carry on with my life. I started taking art classes with a well-known local artist. Eventually, I had to stop because I was too tired to make the drive. I saw a few medical type people during that time, but nobody resonated with me or understood how bad the fatigue was. I was so sick of being misunderstood by people or being passed off as if it was all in my head because to them, I looked fine.

In 2015, I hit rock bottom. The fatigue was so bad that making the bed was an all-day event. Walking down the short driveway to the mailbox was unthinkable. I was extremely upset with my circumstance and thought, "What's the sense of sticking around if I'm going to feel like complete crap all the freaking time? Who the hell do I need to be here for anyway?" In the course of 7 years I lost my mom, dad, grandmother, my husband's grandmother, my father-in-law, and both my dogs. The house was dirty because I didn't have the energy to clean it or keep it organized. Small piles started creeping up in the bedroom where I spent most of my time. I couldn't read books or work on my writing because I couldn't focus on the words. Surely, I wasn't making my husband happy because I never felt like doing anything. He's a great guy, honest and hard-working, he wouldn't have any problem finding another partner.

I started to think of ways of how I would do it. Hanging myself wasn't an option, too many things to think about logistically being only 4'11." Slitting my wrists; I didn't want anyone to have to clean up blood. Maybe I'll over dose on sleeping pills. That seemed like the best way. I could play some calming music. I was so freaking tired that sleeping shouldn't be a problem at all! Perfect. It was settled. No specific date yet. I didn't sleep at all that night and by the next morning I was crying uncontrollably. Barely able to form a sentence, I called my friend who is a therapist. I confessed to her about my thoughts; she demanded that I come see her immediately. "But I'm in my pajamas." I said. "I don't give a rat's ass about your pajamas, get down here."

she said. I explained everything to her: my frustrations with my health and life, my losses, and my bad thoughts. I have never cried that hard in my life. I was embarrassed. I was a successful, well-known business woman who received several awards over the past few years. I was a published writer and columnist. I was thin, pretty, and the "IT" girl in the room that everyone wanted to be around because I was positive, full of energy, and fun. And now it had come to this. She sat patiently and listened. When I was done, she said, "This is what we are going to do. We are going to make a plan for you." For the next hour we sat together and came up with a strategy, a step-by-step if you will of what I would do next. I will never forget that day.

Part of the plan was to make an appointment with a naturopathic doctor in the Springfield, MA area. Putting aside my thoughts about all this, I made the appointment. The doctor ordered bloodwork and determined I had Chronic Fatigue Syndrome, adrenal exhaustion, and the Epstein Barr Virus. I was happy to finally get a diagnosis (so I thought) and she sent me home with a bag full of supplements. I worked with her for a year and a half. In 2016, I decided that I had not experienced a significant change, so I parted ways with the doctor.

In 2017, the fatigue came back with a vengeance. My eyes started bothering me, I gained weight, experienced numbness in my hands, my hair was thinning, I lost part of my eyebrows, I was experiencing night sweats, and I had occasional panic attacks. I was unable to read books or work on my writing because I couldn't focus on the words. I was too tired to work on my art. I stopped attending networking events and meeting friends for coffee because I was worried about driving. I stepped down from all the boards I volunteered for. I worried about traveling because I didn't have the energy to pack.

A friend told me about a naturopathic doctor in West Hartford, CT who had success with patients complaining about fatigue. I made an appointment and gathered my medical records and test results. I put together a timeline of who I had seen, when I saw them, and what they said. As soon as I met the doctor I knew I was in the right place. "You should have had seen a significant difference by now; don't worry, we are going to get to the bottom of all this." he said. I felt validated and trust me, I was going to make sure he kept his word. The results of my bloodwork really told a story. I tested positive again for the Epstein Barr Virus, my adrenals were in full-blown exhaustion, and all my "levels" were very low. He also tested for Lyme Disease using the Western Blot through IGNEX and it came back positive. I was annoyed that my primary care doctor didn't find the Lyme Disease but I was told it was because he kept issuing the wrong type of test. The first naturopath I saw didn't even test for it. The naturopath sent me home with lots of herbs and supplements. I had to use mini Altoid containers to organize them because the pill boxes at the drug store weren't big enough.

Currently it's 2018. I'm feeling better but I still have a way to go. I continue to work with the naturopath and have seen good results. My adrenals and other levels are back to where they need to be. I also sought the advice from an infectious disease doctor in Longmeadow, MA and have come to like and respect the work that she does. I see both doctors on a regular basis. I still experience fatigue, eye strain, numbness in my hands, and recently started getting leg pain. I also know that as the Lyme Disease dies off, my symptoms may get worse. However, with that said, I have more good days now and my hair and eyebrows are growing back.

I'm starting to be more open about my Lyme experience and it's interesting to get reactions from people. They want me to try their supplement, drink their juice, rub this oil or that, eat kale, drink tea. Whatever. When I tell certain people that I decided to take antibiotics I get the "look," as if antibiotics have no place in the healing process; an odd and stubborn stance considering the millions who have been saved with antibiotics. People simply do not comprehend the magnitude and complexity of this disease, and that whatever helps to alleviate its symptoms is a welcome relief.

In the process of all this my life has changed dramatically. Sadly, many friends and business connections have since disappeared or can't be bothered to call or check in. I've had to learn to be more particular about what I want to do with my time and who I want to spend it with. I'm slowly finding new business connections and making new friends. We adopted two Scottish Terriers, Fannie and Farley. They are my personal healthcare agents. They talk to me and make me smile and snuggle with me to keep my painful legs warm. They keep me grounded. I have a friend that lives in Florida, she texts me every day or so to see how I'm doing. I have another friend who is a trainer and I pay her to walk me like a dog. She is a great listener. I have a couple of friends that offer to drive whenever I want to shop or go to a networking event. My husband does all the cooking and grocery shopping and drives me all over the place. Throughout this journey I have been able to maintain my Clutter Doctor and Holistic Healing businesses with patient and caring clients and without compromising who I am as a person or businesswoman. Yesterday I drove 45 minutes to the mall to shop for an upcoming trip. It felt so free to be able to do that. For all this I am grateful.

If you are reading this book because you have Lyme

Disease or think you may have it, my advice is to stay strong and keep investigating all avenues of healthcare to find what works for you. Don't give up! If you are reading this book because someone you know has Lyme Disease, call them, text them, send them notes, offer rides, cook for them, clean for them, visit them, just offer something. It's the thought of you making the suggestion that counts. They need your support!

The other day my husband told me I looked good. These days I feel like the only heads I turn are those of the dogs. But what he said after that really made me happy, "You have a twinkle in your eye that I haven't seen in a long time."

Carleen Eve Fischer Hoffman is the owner of The Clutter Doctor Inc., an award-winning professional organizing business dedicated to helping clients gain control and balance.

Carleen's long work days led her to discover Reiki and

inspired her to open Carleen Hoffman Holistic Healing serving people and pets.

Carleen resides in East Longmeadow, Massachusetts with her husband Brad and their two Scotties, Fannie and Farley. When she's awake, she enjoys writing and creating art, shopping for vintage jewelry, and coffee with friends.

Carleen welcomes questions about her story at carleen@carleenhoffman.com
East Longmeadow, MA

Social Media Public Announcement

By Elise Bugala

I have felt like absolute crap for the last couple of weeks (I don't know if its a Lyme flare or what)... and on top of that I finally found a physical therapist who knows how to help me and I'm not sure I'm going to be able to continue going because I react to the cleaning chemicals or air fresheners they use in the clinic. So it's kind of counter productive because when I leave the place with a migraine, dizziness, crushing fatigue, and nausea that lasts for days its makes it impossible for me to do my home exercises....Or really give it my all when I'm there, which is obviously very counter productive.

I have a million other things going on with my health and its just so much that I don't even know where to begin with treatment. It seems like if I treat one thing it makes another thing worse. I just feel like the last year or so I stopped getting better and I've been declining pretty rapidly.

I have not only been feeling physically sick but also it's

really hard emotionally. Honestly being so disabled has left me feeling like a horrible person. I feel like I can't do anything for anyone, including myself. I can't commit to anything because i never know how I'm going to feel and when I have to cancel something (which usually I'd rather push through and suffer than cancel) I feel like I'm failing and disappointing everyone.

I'm not a good friend because I can never do anything fun with people since I'm allergic to the outside world. Also, school... that's kind of a sore subject but here it is: I am 19 years old have not graduated yet. I've tried everything there is to try school wise and the bottom line is I'm too sick. I'm too sick to even get treatment to not be sick anymore. So at this point a diploma isn't even my top priority anymore. I get all kinds of judgment for that and I guess that's fair... I know its out of love. People are just worried about my future and want the best for me and I appreciate that. But, I already know that I need education to succeed in life; I know that and that's what makes it so terrifying. There are so many things I would like to do with my life, I have career goals and dreams. But right now I don't know what I'm going to do with my life, because at this point I'm not even sure when ill be healthy enough to have a life.

As terrifying and sad as that is for me I am honestly more heartbroken that I don't have the energy to do things for others. I see need in the world and I see opportunity to help and I'm not physically capable of doing anything.

I trained my dog to be a therapy dog but I can only take her for visits once a week and I'm even having a hard time keeping up with that (I've been really thankful for all the snow days that my schools have had on Fridays). I feel like in a way I'm even failing my her. She put in the work to become a therapy dog and I cant even bring her to places to do the job she's worked so hard to have.

Then to top it all off I woke up this morning with horrible pain in my right eye and after an emergency eye doctor visit (thank God I have the best eye doctor in the world) it turns out I injured my cornea and there's a hole in it. I got eye drops to prevent infection and It should heal up within a few days. So its not a huge deal... but like c'mon I just cant seem to catch a break.

Why am I posting this???

Two reasons: I need some prayer and I need some compassion. I really don't like talking about my health. It's not a happy subject and I like to stay positive when talking to others. It makes people uncomfortable to hear bad news, and honestly I don't want to think about it either.

Sometimes it feels good to pretend I'm normal so that I don't have to deal with the reality of my illness. But that's not really fair to anybody... I'm learning that a little honesty goes a long way. I know its kind of frowned upon to "air your dirty laundry" on social media, but I have been lying to a lot of people. So, Facebook is the easiest way for me to let everyone know. Plus, typing it out is easier for me because like I said I don't like to talk about it. (Sorry if we just met or you don't actually know me in person, I'm not trying to freak you out but if you're going to know me... I guess this is what you need to know about me). I don't want you all to pity me but I do feel that you deserve to know what's going on. Its not fair for you to think I don't want to be your friend because we never talk or hangout, or that I don't care about you because I "make excuses" or have to cancel plans. I care about you all and I think you deserve to know what I'm going through so you don't think its a personal problem with you. Also, its easy for me to be deeply hurt and resentful when people make comments about certain subjects (i.e. you're too smart to not be in school, that I lack ambition, that I'm a drama queen, and any other ignorant thing that people have said to me) but if I'm pretending to be healthy while saying I can't do "x y or z" then I have no right to be resentful for you reacting to the information I have given you.

I know I'm smart, I know we'll figure it out eventually, and I know that God has a plan for my life. I have hope and I have faith. Knowing that God is with me gives me peace and makes everything so much easier to get through. I know he holds my future a I know he will use this all for good. I still love life and I try to find joy in every situation.

Really the hardest part of chronic illness is dealing with people who don't understand... and I'm not asking you to understand. I know that unless you've been through something yourself you can't really understand it.... And that's ok.

I'm really not trying to complain (ok...so yeah, I was kinda complaining about the cornea thing... you can pity me for that... its awful!) I'm just putting this all out there so that I can hopefully help ease the strain that has been put on some of my relationships. I kind of found it easier to just distance myself from people then to be honest with them or try to get them to understand, like I said a little honestly goes a long way.

If you made it to the end, thank you for caring enough to read it all... I know this was a little long and a little too "real" for social media.

STORIES FROM CAREGIVERS

Lyme Mom

I couldn't believe my ears. It was May, at the end of 11th grade for my daughter and her guidance counselor just said, "You'll never make it into any college."

Who says stuff like that? And to a kid?

It had ben a rough year. She took her classes online because she couldn't attend school.

High school hadn't gone the way I had envisioned for my beautiful, smart daughter. Entering 11th grade she had been slated to take multiple Advanced Placement courses, including Calculus.

But the fall of 10th grade changed all that.

She had gone to volunteer with her school to clean up a local parks and recreation area and she came home saying she had been bitten by something behind her ear. It looked like an extra big mosquito bite, and she said it felt more like a bee sting. We didn't think much more about it until December when she started complaining that she was dizzy and missed school for 2 weeks because she couldn't stand up.

I took her to my Lyme doctor because I remembered that bite, but my very own Lyme doctor told me that I was being a paranoid Lyme mom because I had Lyme myself and thought everything was Lyme. He adamantly said my daughter's symptoms weren't Lyme. Not wanting to be that paranoid weirdo, I let it drop.

I wish I had persisted. I mean, what's it to him if I pay for the Igenex lab test?

Her ear started to bleed regularly.
She was tired all the time.
She got dizzy.
We went to the ENT and they gave her drops and told me that she must be poking her ear with her finger in the middle of the night.

By summer her face was numb – her extremities too.

The family doctor told us that she had no idea and if it didn't resolve that we were to go to the emergency room. Guess where we were by the next day?

You would've thought a big famous University hospital could have helped and diagnosed her correctly, but you see, the don't believe in Lyme Disease as a real thing. Our state somehow isn't a state with Lyme?

Instead, they brought in a pediatric psychologist and decided she was just over "stressed" by the situation at her dad's, my ex-husband's house. They scheduled a follow up, released us after a long night of testing, lots of tears and this nothing diagnosis.

Thank God our primary care doctor ordered a Lyme test, unbeknownst to me. My daughter was CDC positive and I found out when the county called wanting to know where she had been. Had she been out of the state? Are you sure? Remember, they think that Lyme doesn't exist here. I guess they were confused how she could have Lyme while never leaving the state.

Senior year, my daughter desperately wanted to be back in school. She's an extrovert and being cooped up and not able to go out and be social or be with friends was depressing her.

I got her a 504. Her friend read her English book to her because she couldn't concentrate or comprehend (and she said my voice grated her nerves). But the biggest problem was that no one understood. The kids didn't believe she was truly sick and the teachers didn't think she needed any accommodations.

She was supposed to get a stool to sit on in choir, but she never did. I had it out with that teacher and his response was, "YOU are the only one who ever brings up that she's sick. She never says anything!"

Hello?

Contrary to popular belief, Lyme kids (and I would guess most chronically ill children) do not want to be singled out. They don't want to be known as sickies. They want to be seen as normal. They complain very little about their issues, muddle through their pain, and if they do say something, they're generally misunderstood which is the exact reason they stop bringing it up.

Lyme kids just want to be able to participate in the normal things that other kids do like sports, theater, special events, and prom. They'll do themselves in for weeks afterwards just for one chance at having a normal kid's day.

The problem is that their friends only see them when they're up to putting on that fake, "I'm okay," smile or there's something happening that they just don't want to miss.

You don't see them out when they feel so bad they can't stand seeing the light.
You don't see them when the pain is so bad they're curled up in a ball crying in bed.
You don't see them when they don't have the energy to even get up the stairs.

I was determined to make the final year of school easier

for my daughter so during orientation for 12th grade, I walked into the school with pamphlets (https://www.lymediseaseassociation.org/about-lyme/lyme-kids-a-schools/586-abcs-of-lyme-disease-lda-pamphlet) about Lyme Disease to explain to the teachers. I even wrote up a cover letter with further explanations and statistics. I have no idea if they read it after I talked to them, but at least I had the short chat during our time together. I explained why she had a 504.

It didn't help.

The choir teacher never gave her that stool. He actually made her lift heavy stage equipment to help set up and she would come home exhausted, in pain and crying because she had tried so hard to just "suck it up" and do it. No matter how much I told her to say something, she just didn't want to call attention to herself for being sick because the kids were already giving her a hard time.

Her school guidance counselor never believed there was anything wrong with her. The superintendent never returned my call. None of the teachers ever followed the 504.

And guess what? She did get into college. I wish I could tell that guidance counselor what I thought of her. My daughter still remembers her words.

But guess what else?

Everything repeated itself in college. They didn't believe she was sick. In fact, at her school, attendance was part of your grade. If you were sick and missed class, you could fail purely by attendance even if your grade was still good enough to pass, even with a doctor's note.

Her IBS (Irritable Bowl Syndrome) got so bad she was constantly in the bathroom or doubled up on the floor, yet she was required to at least show up to class and be there at the end of class even if she left in between. This was a Christian school too!

Her guidance counselor in college asked why she

needed help and denied giving her any, even with the 504 still in place. She had finally asked for the help she needed and was told to, "Just try harder!"

She visited the hospital every year except her last, but only because she realized they couldn't help her so it wasn't worth the expense.

We did one good thing in December of 2016 during Christmas break. We decided to spend the holidays doing UBI (Ultraviolet Blood Irradiation) treatments. We had tried so much already – from the antibiotics, to the homeopathics to herbs and rife machine, but the inconsistency of treatment during highs school and college wasn't really helping the Lyme. This was our last big shot.

Ten sessions later, and thousands of dollars of uninsured medical costs later, my daughter had her blood cleaned with UBI. It has definitely helped her to be sick less often though it didn't completely fix her.

I'm happy to say she persisted in her studies and stayed

committed to getting her degree. She graduates this year with a major and a minor (and a boyfriend).

As a mom, I hate to see my child suffer and I'm also proud of what she's accomplished. Despite all the ups and downs and things she thought I might be disappointed with because she didn't get that A grade, I'm happy that future seems brighter and that she's learned how to better cope with Lyme Disease.

Where is my Casserole?

A Parent's Perspective of Lyme Disease

by Becky Bugala

I have been mulling over what to write and decided to be brutally honest.

My husband and I have three wonderful kids, and two of them have Lyme and co-infections. It stinks!

We have watched them suffer for 16 years. They have only been diagnosed for five years. One kid mainly has had psychiatric symptoms, and the other has the "full Monty" of chronic pain, fatigue, brain fog, gastric distress, dizziness, Ad nauseum – literally!

Their illnesses have robbed them of their health, education, friends, and sometimes family. In addition to their symptoms, they have dealt with misdiagnosis, disbelief, an utter lack of help from traditional medical professionals, leaving us all feeling frustrated and helpless!

It has been a very lonely journey for our family. I have often said, "If the kids had cancer, the entire community would rally around us." There would be fundraisers, offers to help galore, and…casseroles! "Where is my casserole?!" She said, only half kidding.

I have heard that there are lessons in everything and here are some I've learned on this journey:

- We are doing the best we can, and we can do better.
- We cycle through the grief process as the illness waxes and wanes.
- Life is lived one day at a time, and even the worst day ends.
- There is always hope! People can and do improve, and go into remission.
- Gratitude is the best remedy for fear, hopelessness, self-pity and sadness.
- Prayer is imperative for us, and we fall into our father's arms daily.
- Finally, this is not what we envisioned for our children, yet they are living life, finding joy and humor (sometimes very dark) moment by

moment.

We may be lonely and sometimes heartbroken, yet are not alone in our suffering. I believe that they will continue to be courageous and inspiring as they search for healing.

When Your Children Live with Lyme Too

by Anonymous

As a Mommy you pray for a healthy baby. You count fingers and toes and wait for that first cry indicating that everything will be alright. Our children were born perfectly healthy by definition. They met milestones, ate well, slept well, and are the most loveable sweet children you could meet.

Except, that something didn't seem quite right. They would get the shivers constantly, even with it wasn't chilly. One would scream out in devastating pain randomly that her eye hurt so incredibly bad. It would take a warm washcloth, rocking, and singing for about ten minutes to get her back to feeling well enough to get down.

My other daughter would get out of bed in the morning and immediately fall to the floor at a two years old exclaiming that her legs hurt too bad to walk. Thankfully for mothers intuition, always trust that above anything else, and Igenex speciality lab testing, we got out answer. They too had Lyme Disease.

The only thing worse than living with Lyme Disease yourself, is knowing your children have to live with it too. As a mother you don't want life to be anymore difficult for your children than it has to be. I cried for days, mourning the loss of health and being terribly scared. Then it happened, God send me a message that he chose me to be their Mommy because I get it.

We have so much fun at our house! We laugh, smile, read, play games, take trips when we are well, but most of all we know what we have to do to keep our Lyme Disease in check.

We have strict diets, strict bedtimes, schedules that need careful monitoring, and just some days of rest that are needed more for them then a normal child. But, they are treating and improving. We are going to make it.

Above all, we have each other. A special bond that goes deeper than mother and daughter, but that is brought about because we truly know each others pain and body. I pray every day and night for a cure for Lyme Disease for my darlings. Nothing would be a bigger blessing. However, we choose to take advantage of our good days, rest on our bad days, and above all love each other through it, because Lyme Disease is not for the weak.

My girls are pretty tough cookies and I am in awe of how they handle it all with grace and dignity, even at such a young age. They will make it, we will make it, and together we will fight for a cure for this awful disease.

Why Don't They Understand?

by Alana Stamper

The school was calling again. It was a rotation of which of my children they were calling about. They were all missing too many days school. They said they'd contact truancy and even CPS even though I had a had a doctor note explaining.

Didn't they understand? My kids have Lyme disease.

And I do too.

I got bit by the tick when I was 6. I remember feeling sick all the time, tired, I wondered what it felt like to not feel sick like my friends. It started with constant kidney and bladder infections. It's also the explanation for why I was constantly pulling muscles, getting hurt and breaking bones. Thing was, I didn't find out until I was 34 that I had chronic Lyme Disease. My doctors were too confused by my symptoms and I was misdiagnosed with lupus, MS, colitis, optical and Trigeminal neuralgia, possible seizures but nothing they did ever eased my symptoms.

I have a doctor for Lyme.
I have a neurologist for Lyme.
I have an Neuro eye specialist for Lyme.

Between juggling my own Lyme issues and doctors visits, I have to take my 5 kids ages 3 through 16 to all their activities and doctor appointments too. As much as we try to coordinate them, it doesn't always work out. I feel like I'm at the doctor's office more than my own home, and way more than I'm able to be in my own bed!

After that year with the kids being sick so often, I finally decided to homeschool them. While that's hard, what's harder as a mom is watching your kids struggle or not be able to participate in activities because their Lyme symptoms are flaring.

If they were better at testing and diagnosing this disease I could've treated during all five of my pregnancies and reduced the risk of my kids getting it greatly.

The symptoms my kids experience the most are: tired all the time, muscle pain, joint pain, headaches, anxiety, sleep problems, hard time concentrating, they get sick easily and stay sick longer.

The symptoms I personally experience the most are: constant migraines, muscle spasms and weakness, pulled muscles and tendons, still brake bones easily, vertigo, joint pain, nerve pain, horrible immune system, extremely tired, sleep problems due to pain, migraines and muscle spasms, rashes, a constant growing list of food allergies and allergic reactions almost daily (hives and throat swells up). I also have extreme amount of stress for what having this disease does to us financially.

And I take care of a family of 7 with 3 dogs!

Here's what I wish people understood about kids with Lyme: when you're born with it, it means they know no different and smile even thought they're in tremendous pain. Can you imagine never ever having experienced a pain free day of living? Can you imagine if that was your norm? That's what Lyme kids go through.

And they learn to fake it through their day. I'm blessed because my kids have happy, smiling dispositions – I don't know how I got so lucky! The problem with it is that sometimes they don't tell me everything about what's going on because they know I'm sick too and they don't want to overburden me.

I think the hardest thing for a mom to hear is that a teacher or someone else might think a child is lazy because they have Lyme. They're not lazy – they're beyond exhausted. I know for myself that as soon as I wake up, I wish it was time to go to bed again. Imagine never waking up refreshed for decades of your life … then try to function well throughout your day.

And while we suffer, I hold on to the hope that we will all be healed one day and be able to live the vibrant lives that every loving mother wishes for her children.

LYME

by Michael Gould

I'm not a writer, I'm just an average guy, a husband, a father, that has experienced good and not so good things through this journey that we have been on. I do however, want to first and foremost state that there were many many times that I blew it. Many more than I wish to remember.

The challenge and difficulty come when you watch a person go from being full of life to someone that doesn't have the ability to get out of bed and felt like she was a burden to those around her; and then back to someone that represents a relative likeness of the person you knew at the beginning.

It's in those times that you find yourself faced with things that you have never faced before. What do you say, what do you not say, what do you do, what do you not do, how do you help, is it the right help, is your help even wanted, do you leave them alone, do you not leave them alone, how long with this last, will it ever be different, and will the person you once knew ever be back?

L- Life, Love, Longing

She was full of life. She seemed to never stop, always doing something. She had this way about her that she wanted to constantly be learning or experiencing something new. If you could do something she felt she could do it too.

Early on in our relationship we went to Virginia on a weeklong ski trip. We enjoyed our time together skiing, eating of course, and just being together. While on the ski hill one of those days we found a place that someone had made a small ski jump. So, I went over it and after stopping, turning, and checking to see if she was still with me the next thing I see is her going over the jump too. Well, let's just say after that we needed to go get her new skis. She was fine, but off to the ski shop we went.

She wasn't much of an outdoors kind of person and

really doesn't like the outdoors at all. But, if it was something that interested me she would do it just because she loved me. One of earliest camping trips including taking our boat along and going fishing on Saginaw Bay. It wasn't her thing, but again she did it because she wanted to be with me.

Once the disease started to take over her body she quickly became a shell of what she once was. She was not the same person that I had watched do the things she did and was constantly on the move. Her time now for the most part was spent in bed feeling terrible. What happened to that person?

There was a feeling of missing my partner. There was a sense of mourning that it appeared I would never have my wife back; a longing to have her back.

Y- Why?

Why her? Why was this happening to us? Why was she so angry for what seemed like all the time? The littlest things or even what appeared to be nothing sparked what I called "jumping to level 10" with no warning.

Why does she feel like a burden? There were times that the combination of symptoms, wondering if this is what life was going to be like until the end, and adding in this feeling of being a burden she would just wish GOD would take her.

Why did she wish that? It was very hard to watch and hear, but I would try to tell her that GOD had a plan for her and he was going to use this experience to help someone else. That was easy for me to say, I wasn't the one in the bed. I did truly believe that.

M- Mother, Marriage, Me

She couldn't go on the kid's school trips or attend the school parties. Each time one would come up she would just cry knowing she was missing out. What seemed to bother her even more was that her kids were growing up without a mother.

What was amazing however, is that no matter how she

felt she would ensure that there was a meal on the table for dinner. The effect of doing just that one task would put her right back to bed for the evening. It was very draining on her.

I don't wish this on any family, but if there is a bright spot in all of this now that the kids are older is that they very independent and can do many things that their friends have never been asked to do.

Where is my wife? She's here in the house, but the person I knew; the person I married isn't here.

The anger and rage would seem to come from nowhere. It wouldn't stop. From my perspective I thought I was being understanding, trying to listen to what she was saying, trying to be empathetic to the symptoms she was describing. But looking back at it now I didn't have a clue to what she was going thru.

I wasn't in her shoes living with what she was. I've been nauseous, I've been tired, and I've had headaches, body aches, pains, dizziness. But the difference was I didn't have them all at the same time, constantly reminding me that they were there, and never going away.

Why didn't she see that I was trying to help? Or so I thought I was. The problem is it wasn't the help that she really needed. Of course, taking care of the kids, making sure the leftovers from dinner were put away, making sure the dishes were done, getting the kids to their activities, etc were all helping, but it wasn't the help that she really needed.

What do I do now? How do we move forward? What is life going to look like? What I should have done looking back was recognized the most important thing she needed was for me to just hold her and let her know everything was going to be all right.

E- Energy, End

Being bedridden for most of the day and not having the energy (or feeling well enough) to get out of bed she would turn the internet; spending hours researching and researching and researching what would help her get better.

She learned so much that her conversations with the doctors were on a level that it seemed she knew more than they did about the disease; the symptoms. And you know what, she did know more.

She tried all different kinds of protocols, none were pharma (prescription drugs); she did it all natural. And over time it started to work, it started to change how she was feeling, she was able to get out of bed for longer and longer periods of time, and the rage/anger started to subside.

And after these number of years I started to see that person coming back. The person that wouldn't let something like this win. The person that showed me the energy she had early on.

There have been many ups and downs in this journey, but I strongly believe that the experiences we go through prepare us to be able to help someone else in the future. She has been able to share her journey, share what worked for her, and give hope to others.

The Political Madness of Chronic Lyme Disease

by Lori Dennis

I am not a microbiologist, a medical doctor or a public health official. I am not a journalist, an academic researcher or a politician.

I am a mother whose adult son fell ill several years ago with a 'mysterious' cascade of symptoms. An illness that took over his life like an unsympathetic terrorist and forced us to become expert scientists and sleuths.

When after eighteen months of witnessing our son suffer, and after consulting twenty different medical specialists in New York City all of whom were somehow not able to determine the root cause of his unrelenting symptoms, it became our job to figure it out. And figure it out we did.

This was just the start of our medical odyssey. Our entrée into an alternate universe we've come to know as Lymeland. A place where tens of millions around the globe are suffering. A place where very few doctors, public health officials, politicians, and journalists are listening. A place that, no matter where we turn, we are presented by a steel wall of denial and mistruths, preventing men, women and children in eighty countries from getting the medical care they desperately need and deserve.

Navigating our son's chronic Lyme disease has been one of the most difficult journeys of our lives. When you or a loved one become ill and you cannot find a medical professional to help you determine why, and the burden then falls on you to navigate this 'do-it-yourself' disease, you are left with no choice but to learn and learn fast.

You search and you search. You read anything and everything in sight. You ask a lot of questions. You listen to what the so-called 'trusted experts' are saying. You listen to what the so-called 'fringe experts' are saying. You are forced to trust your gut, your intuition, and your own personal experience to determine where to go and what to do.

For several years now, chronic Lyme disease has been a hyperfocus, to say the least. I've spent countless hours digging, deciphering, reading, researching, analyzing, and inquiring. Several years helping my son navigate his illness while bearing witness to a bottomless pit of global human suffering by millions who have been rendered voiceless, and left to suffer in silence.

You see, not only is chronic Lyme disease itself incredibly complex, ugly and parasitic, so are the medical politics driving it. It is the twisted and mountainous medical politics that compel me to fight—seeking justice from a system that has somehow gone terribly wrong.

The decades-old falsehoods, disinformation, greed, profit, ego, and arrogance driving this 'political disease' have turned Lyme into a universal experience of gaslighting, sick shaming, blaming and discrediting of millions of patients worldwide. World-over, Lyme sufferers in response to their cries for help are told by their doctors that they can't possibly have chronic Lyme disease because…

"There is no such thing as chronic Lyme…Chronic Lyme disease is the 'disease du jour'…There is no Lyme in this country, city, town, region…Ticks don't cross the border…You didn't go hunting in the highlands of Scotland, did you?…If you didn't see the tick, you can't have Lyme…If you didn't see the bulls-eye rash, you don't have Lyme…Your blood tests were indeterminate, negative, false positive…A round of antibiotics and you'll be as good as new…When did you get your medical degree?…Google is not medical school…You don't have an elevated white blood cell count so you can't have Lyme…You don't have arthritis so you can't have Lyme… I don't know anything about Lyme disease but I can tell you, you don't have it…You look too good to be that sick…These are just normal signs of aging…Everyone feels tired…Get fresh air and exercise…You're depressed…You're stressed…You're just feeling anxious…Stop dwelling on your problems…Think positively…Try praying…I'll refer you to a psychiatrist…An antidepressant and therapy should do the trick."

These inane pronouncements made by doctors daily are causing Lyme sufferers to feel like they're crazy, lazy, overdramatizing, misinterpreting, histrionic, malingering, and just plain wrong. The best doctors can do, it seems, is tell their patients that it's 'all in their heads' and then offload them to a psychiatrist for meds and therapy.

I can assure you that chronic Lyme disease is very real, the suffering that Lyme patients are forced to endure is very real, and the number of people affected by the disease—both directly and indirectly—is growing exponentially, while the medical establishment continues to do very little to address it.

In the years that we've been held captive in Lymeland, a place that closely resembles The Walking Dead, here is what I've come to understand about chronic Lyme disease:

- It is a global pandemic.

- The medical 'powers that be' are not taking any

meaningful measures to stop this pandemic from growing—and it is growing more and more each day, in more than eighty countries. By 2020, 80% of Canadians, for example, will be exposed to ticks. So yes, you and your loved ones could be next.

•   Research tells us that this disease can be transmitted not just by ticks but by other vectors such as mosquitoes, fleas, flies and bedbugs, as well as congenitally, via breastfeeding, blood transfusions and organ donations.

•   Millions of men, women and children around the globe are suffering in horrid, inhumane, unimaginable ways, every single day and most do not have access to medical care.

•   Most mainstream doctors stand in firm denial of this illness, insisting that there is no such thing, that your symptoms are all in your head, that you are suffering from conversion disorder or some such psychiatric illness.

•   Chronic Lyme disease is not an infectious disease

but a B Cell AIDS. A post-sepsis, immunosuppressive illness caused by shed fungal outer surface proteins (OspA) of a spirochete, which detonate the immune system and open the floodgates for opportunistic infections, bacteria, parasites, mold, retroviruses and herpes viruses such as EBV and HHV6.

• Contrary to what we are told, this disease is not driven by spirochetal persistence. That is not what keeps people sick. It is OspA—a fungal endotoxin—causing global immune suppression that keeps chronic Lyme sufferers from recovering their health. And too few know it.

• To make matters worse, LYMErix, the Lyme vaccine of the late 1990's was made with OspA which rendered people sick with chronic Lyme disease.

In 2002, GlaxoSmithKline decided to withdraw LYMErix from the market citing poor market performance and blaming negative press coverage when, in fact, the real pressure was coming from the mounting number of lawsuits due to severe adverse reactions.

- In short, chronic Lyme disease cannot be prevented by a vaccine. Why? Because spirochetes shed fungal antigens creating a disease of immunosuppression. You cannot vaccinate against Lyme any more than you can vaccinate against tuberculosis or syphilis. You cannot vaccinate against a fungal endotoxin. It can't be done.

- But wait! There's a new Lyme vaccine in the pipeline. This new money-maker could be the reason the CDC finally decided to increase the 'official' number of Lyme cases from 30,000 to 300,000 practically overnight. This new vaccine is likely the next golden goose for who have puppeteered this global medical holocaust and pervasive denial for more than 40 years. Buyer beware!!!

- And, finally, here is the reason for this decades-old war: The Bayh-Dole Act of 1980 fundamentally changed the way that the U.S. commercialized technology by enabling universities, non-profit research institutions and small businesses to patent, license and retain title to groundbreaking discoveries. Driven by this new medical heyday and unprecedented profit incentive, the orchestrators of the 1994 Dearborn Conference falsified the definition of chronic Lyme disease admitting only those cases with an 'arthritic knee type illness' (15%) vs. an immunosuppressive, neurological illness (85%) in order to bring a Lyme vaccine to market. They knew that they couldn't sell a vaccine for the immunosuppressive cases which made up the vast majority of chronic Lyme sufferers. So they threw out the real case definition and narrowed it to fit their vaccine model. This is why, to this day, doctors tell us there is 'no such thing as chronic Lyme', that it's 'a mere nuisance arthritic condition', and that a few days or at most a few weeks of antibiotics and you should be as good as new.

This deeply entrenched denial of chronic Lyme disease—driven by the falsehoods disseminated by mainstream medicine long ago —is the root of the madness and the reason that chronic Lyme sufferers are victimized:

- By the disease itself.
- By doctors who turn their backs.
- By loved ones who roll their eyes and walk away.

- By insurance companies who refuse to provide coverage.
- By the CDC and the IDSA who together insist that chronic Lyme disease does not exist.

When you listen to the deniers of this disease, and there are plenty of them, ask yourself this:Is it really possible that millions of once healthy, active individuals, the world over, are faking their illness, suffering daily beyond the pale, and are participating in some kind of mass delusion? Is it really possible that they are pretending to be sick because they have no better life plan than to become housebound, infirm, isolated, and penniless, and looking for some kind of perverse attention with no perceivable payoff?

I urge you to investigate this madness. Our collective hope is that one day the rest of the world will become as outraged as we are by this medical travesty.

This madness needs to stop. Sadly though, as the saying goes, most probably won't get it until they actually 'get it'. Because the truth of the matter is far too dark and hideous for the human psyche to truly comprehend.

In the meantime, along with my many colleagues in the trenches of Lymeland, I will keep talking, writing, educating, protesting, petitioning, and fighting…while continuing to let the light seep through the cracks until the day this medical travesty transforms into the most extraordinary of human triumphs. I hope that day comes soon.

Lori Dennis, MA, RP is a Registered Psychotherapist and the author of LYME MADNESS, named #1 NEW RELEASE in Immune System Health on Amazon. LYME MADNESS is available on Amazon. For more information, go to www.loridennisonline.com.

She's Too Little, It Can't be Lyme

by Jillian Burgess

So when I vocalize about Lyme disease a lot it's because of May 12, 2015.

My then almost 12 month old was playing in our backyard in downtown in the CITY of Appleton. She was bit by a bug on her arm- twice in same spot. I'm 100% convinced mosquito but will never know. We never saw the bug that bit her.

That night in her bath I noticed it. Just looked like a normal mosquito bite. Then over the next 10 days it changed slowly. I took her in. It was dismissed as a normal bug bite. It wasn't sitting right with me but I said ok. As it changed and changed I brought her in again. I was dismissed again. She also had a rash on her face that I was told it was Impetigo by a local pediatrician who GOOGLED for me while I sat with my baby in her office. She wasn't sure what the bite was but said it was NOT Lyme - just a big bug bite. I knew she was wrong...I just knew it.

3 weeks after -the rash disappeared- bite was gone-symptoms began. High fevers out of no where. Not eating. Back to the doc we go. Was told "some kids just get fevers" "some kids just get sick". I was fuming. I knew just knew it was this bite she had. That night at 2 am my almost 12 month old had a seizure next to me in bed. I heard her clicking and jerking and screamed at my husband to call 911. She was so so hot. Chris frantically grabbed our seizing baby and ran downstairs with her. I screamed at the dispatcher to please get medics here!!! I thought she was dying. My little girl laid there convulsing...eyes rolling to back of head...soundless except for the clicking. When she stopped seizing she threw up. We turned her to her side and the paramedics walked in. She began to cry...thank God. No parent wants to watch their tiny baby seize. I remember just taking the biggest breath...like she's alive she's alive okay okay - It's gut wrenching.

The paramedic held her hot body and tried to console me. She was only in her diaper and we went into that ambulance where I pleaded with them to tell me what's wrong with her. Her temp was 104 in the ambulance. At 3 am I get a talk from the ER Doc how "kids just get seizures sometimes," and "kids just get high fevers sometimes". I felt here docs were failing us. I took home my sick baby. Hurt and scared .... During this she was put on 2 weeks antibiotic. Just in case. I pleaded for longer. She was so ill when I took her to a pediatric dermatologist for the rash on her face. I said could this be Lyme? He said he wasn't sure but if it was his kid he would treat. (Lyme treatment needs minimum of 6-8 weeks). She finished the two weeks and was still sick. Woke up again that following Saturday with high fever. Another high fever!! I was losing hope. She had her second seizure in the pediatricians office while we waited. She seized in front of me, the pediatrician on call, and two nurses. I went to the hall screaming for help. Nurses flooded into the room. After the seizing stopped and she threw up I held her and just sobbed. I felt SO lost. So alone. They decided she needed shot of rochepin in her thighs. They then held her tiny body down and did a catheter and blood sample. I could barely stand .... thought I would pass out. My tiny baby screaming for me and I couldn't help her. I held her as I got the talk again! My head was spinning. " some kids just get sick," and " some kids just get fevers".   Did you know her so called fever taken at that appointment was 98.5??!!!! By this point we had seen 6 medical doctors and 1 pediatric dermatologist. Not one said Lyme except a "maybe" from the pediatric dermatologist. I was told her "rash wasn't red enough"..."the ring wasn't thick enough around the bite" and the rash on her face was just coincidence. Exact words. I was done with these docs. Done.

I had Brynn privately tested through a lab called Igenex. They have the most sensitive testing in the US for Lyme. Waited 3 weeks for results. I opened the results ...positive for Lyme disease. I cried. Mostly cause I was sad but more cause I was relieved that my gut was right. We met with a Lyme literate doctor who took us seriously. We learned what we thought were febrile seizures were more likely the Lyme bacteria attacking her brain. I'm still on the fence with that.....We had 2 months of active -consistent-treatment- antibiotics and herbal drops to help kill the Lyme. I'm so thankful for that man and what he did to help us. I will have to watch

Brynn the rest of her life and pray the Lyme is gone or at least at bay. We will never know. I am vocal because Lyme is scary and misunderstood. These nasty insects can transmit so many diseases. Check your kids your dog yourself etc. Prevention is the only way .... Help out there for Lyme is small and people are dying. Insurances won't cover it and these people fight to live every single day.

Protect yourself #lymediseaseawareness

Jillian Burgess. Mother of two and one furry son. Daughter is a Lyme disease warrior and her son is a Brachial plexus warrior. Stay at home momma. Her kids are her life and she'd do anything for them. Married to her wonderful husband.

My Story

By Kelsey O'Brien

"My first symptoms started back when I was 11 years old. Joint problems and a so-called, unexplained back and rib injury. At the time, we tried every doctor, treatment, medication and pain killer we could think of. It got to the point where nothing affected the excruciating pain I was experiencing, and many doctors had admitted that they couldn't help me. Although my body felt broken, countless X-rays, MRIs, CT scans, blood tests claimed that everything was fine.

For those of you with Lyme know that the journey up until the actual diagnosis is truly a devastating, frustrating and confusing time. Mine happened to be about five years long, BUT I got through it. I finally found that I had Lyme in May of 2013. At the time, I was so relieved. I had an actual diagnosis, started treatment, and finally had an explanation whenever anybody asked what was wrong with me (because no, I wasn't faking it!!).

I thought I was going to get better and all the health complications I had gone through were going to be put in the past. But, because I was so unfamiliar with this illness, at first, what I didn't realize was how crazy the Lyme world really is. A year ago, when I started my senior year, was when Lyme affected me neurologically. Once Lyme gets into your brain, it completely takes over you and your life, and all you can do is watch.

I started developing mental confusion (lack of understanding, focus, concentration). I started noticing the memory loss, blurry vision, chronic fatigue, insane headaches/migraines, as well as the continuous severe joint pains, and other symptoms I'm probably forgetting. I could no longer physically or mentally handle school… or anything else for that matter. I got my PICC line put in back in January, and for the first few months of the IV treatment, I minimally was able to leave bed.

Side story; when I was getting my PICC line put in, the nurse at the hospital was commenting on how I must have been excited I got to miss school….little did he know that I hadn't stepped foot in my school for nearly two months. Just goes to show how people truly don't GET it. Eventually, I was able to get a tutor and got myself to graduate high school. Now, I'm almost 18, and although I'm still sick with many of the same symptoms, I'm not as bad as I once was. I'm going into my ninth month of IV antibiotics as well as the other additional oral antibiotics and medications.

I wrote this song because as tough as it is having a disease, having one that lacks knowledge, research, and understanding from people, including the medical field, is even tougher. I wanted to try and explain what it was like to live with Lyme and how it feels knowing that not everyone believes in it, or is willing to fight for those who are suffering from it.

This illness has changed me and my life in more ways than I ever could have imagined, and I know that there are millions of others out there who are going through the exact same thing, if not much worse.

I hope everyone going through this experience is able to relate to my song and story. We must continue to spread awareness and fight for proper testing, diagnosing, treatment, and most importantly, a cure!"

LYRICS: Lyme World

I never thought I'd be in this world that people don't believe in.

Underestimated, so many suffering and not a cure to be found.

They tell me that I look fine,

But little do they know how bad I feel inside.

I smile through the pain,

Pray that one day this will all go away.

I bet you didn't know

There's a knife in my head,

A boulder going through my back,

Shooting pains down my legs.

I bet you didn't know

Last night I was in tears,

So tired from it all,

I've been fighting for so many years.

Day by day I have no control,

These demons take away

Whatever they want.

I ask myself "why me?"

Because it breaks my heart

That I've had to give up everything.

But I smile through the pain,

Pray that one day they'll believe it's not all in my head.

But I bet you didn't know

I no longer feel like myself.

Physically I'm in pain, mentally I'm in a different world.

I bet you didn't know this disease could go so far,

And I'm just one of many trying not to fall.

I'm trying not to fall.

I never thought I'd be in this world that people don't believe in.

Please believe in me.

Kelsey's song:

https://youtu.be/J3yJePfGugo

Lyme Art Show

by Stephanie Lyskawa

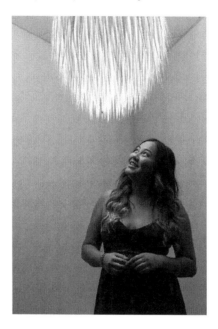

The Waiting Room, a solo show by Stephanie Lyskawa opened on April 24, 2018. The show was in "I" gallery at Azusa Pacific University.

When I was thinking about what I wanted this show to be, I really struggled. An art professor said that this show should be my one thing that I want to say to my peers before I go. For a long time, I didn't know what that was. I was worried that I'd say the wrong thing, not say something good or simply not having anything to say at all. I even struggled with the medium. I primarily work on graphics and take photos but I have a passion for other mediums as well. Most people tell their stories as a recap of their life or a cause they feel passionate about but my life recap and passion went hand in hand and it wasn't something that I wanted to air out.

My Lyme disease diagnosis came in August of 2012. I had gone almost a year without being diagnosed. I've been on this journey for 7 years now. It's weird to think that at one point in my life that I wasn't somewhat sick. It's part of who I am. I tend to stay away from talking about it. It's not because it's hard to talk about, but because if I dwell in it to long I get sad about how much I missed or how much people don't understand or how much and who I had to fight to get my voice heard. I didn't want to fight to get my voice heard in my show and I didn't want others to feel sad about what I went through. So I stayed away from wanting anything having to do with Lyme and art.

Of course that didn't happen. Everything I thought of felt

shallow and boring so I wandered back to Lyme Disease. So what was I going to say about it? I didn't want it to turn into some glorified pity party. Instead, I wanted viewers to come in and leave knowing that even when life throws something difficult your way, that it can still be beautiful. So how was I going to do it?

It all started with photos (of course) but not in the way you might think. I'm talking about photos of my brain. Over the years I've had so many scans of my body that I thought it would be interesting to do something with them. I tinkered with putting photos in the negative space. Because so much of my work revolves around other people, I thought about putting people in that space. Other people just didn't seem appropriate with something so personal though. So I moved to pictures of me and my family, mainly when I was a kid and I didn't have to worry about my Lyme. I wanted to go back and reflect on a time where I was naive about the future.

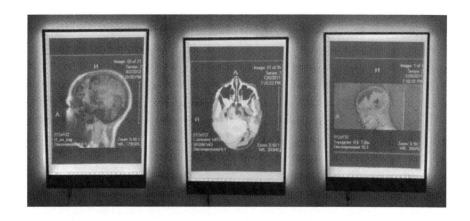

Over the years, I have gathered hundreds of papers of medical records. There wasn't some ah ha moment with what I wanted to do with them. I stumbled on the idea while I was watching a YouTube video about interior design. So I created a light sculpture out of my stack of papers.

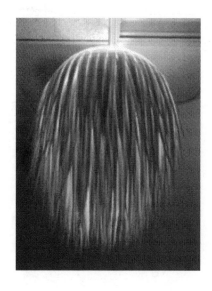

The last pieces for my show are my ceramics. I really love how the clay feels in my hand in the rhythm of the moving circle of the wheel. It's my default happy place where I can block out the world if I need to. My favorite thing to do with the ceramic however is to bend it and manipulate it from its perfect circle to something that has ridges and movement. In it's new form, it turns into something that's far less practical but far more beautiful (in my personal opinion). It's something that was intended to be smooth and even and it's not. It's like me.

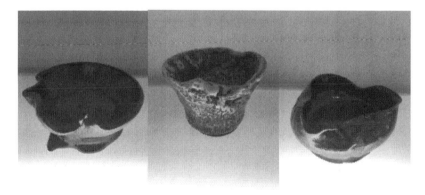

I thought I was going to live this healthy life and I'm not. And its ok. Because while I didn't think I was going to be sick, my Lyme shaped my life into something else - something that is just as beautiful.

LYME WALL OF WARRIORS

Honoring those who fight Lyme Disease

Only .03% (less than ½ of a percent) of 300,000 cases of Lyme per year in the USA is represented with these names!

Abigail Wenger
Adam C Hubers
Alana Stamper
Allison Abernathy
Allison Colla
Ann Gallagher-Aronsen
Annmarie Kampf
Ariel Finck
Ashley Jackson
Aubrey Hines
Austin Cavataio
Barbara Spaulding
Bethany Gillette
Bev Strayer-Grunheid
Brooke Goodgame
Candice Mallicoat
Carleen Eve Fischer Hoffman
Carole Kamerman
Cassidy Colbert
Catherine Spaulding Morales
Celia Lyons
Christopher Cavalotto
Cole Cavataio
Craig Spaulding
Cullan Finck

Dawn Morrison
Debi Sylvia
Denise Northcutt
Dwayne Higdon
Elisabeth Bise
Elise Bugala
Gabbi H.
Gallagher-Aronsen
Gregory J Schnoor
Greta Meyers
Hannah Coughlin
Hannah Spaulding
Holli Crear
Holli V.
Holly Coleman
Imani Young
Jacob Adams
Janet Elizabeth Schmidt Albrecht
Jeanne L Rosario
Jennifer Skender Burns
Jennifer Skender-Burns
Jessica DuMond
Jessica Thomas
Jill Lashua
John Coughlin

Jon Rothberg

Joseph Scuteri

Joy Adams

Julia Deanna Angell Dodds

Kalina Silva

Kari Prince

Kathleen Heath Sullivan Meyer

Kathryn Abernathy

Kerry Windle

Kerry Windle

Khaya Davidson

Kian Silva

Kim Jannick

Kim Luton

Kirsten Albrecht Riehle

Kizzy Crowell

Kory James

Kristina Hartsuck

Larry Maione

Laura Alexandra Grabill

Lauren R.

Lauren White

Laurie Hollander

Laurie Penner

LeeONz

Leslie Davenport-Johnson

Linda Drury

Lisa Dennys

Lois Bunker

Meghan Simkin

Melissa DeMuth

Melissa Fletcher

Michelle Beal

Monika Gotthardt-Marshall

Nicole Rycerz

Niki Baroni Cavataio

Pamela Ammons

Pamela Reardon

Patrick Singhoe

Paula Heaberlin

Rachael Goetz

Rachel Swanson

Riley Johnson

Robert Beasley

Robyn Lamont

Russell Adams

Samuel Bugala

Sarah Ceasar

Sarah Cornish

Sarah Rose

Sonya Finck

Stefanie Wozniak

Susan J Bush

Teri Mitchell

Teri Mitchell

Todd Whiting

Troy Cochran

Wendi R.

Quick Facts: http://www.ilads.org/lyme/lyme-quickfacts.php

This Anthology was compiled by Vickie Gould who was diagnosed with Chronic Lyme Disease in 2009.

ABOUT VICKIE GOULD

Vickie Gould is a certified Law of Attraction business and book coach who has studied under Joe Vitale and is currently coached by Lisa Nichols. Using her signature holistic strategy, she helps her clients go from blank page to best seller, grow their following, help others who are struggling, attract ideal clients, increase their income, and make the worldwide impact that they desire.

Vickie is the author of 7 international best-selling books like *Hit Publish!* and *Standing in the Gap*, and has also helped 59 other entrepreneurs become worldwide best-selling authors. She has been seen on ABC, NBC, CBS, and Fox, was a frequent contributor to HuffPost and Thrive Global, and has previously published an online magazine.

Vickie lives in Michigan with her husband and three

children. She's currently working on an anthology project showcasing entrepreneurs' stories of overcoming adversity, and she is also embarking on a new novel based on stories from her own life.

Join her Facebook Group, Write Your Biz Book for free coaching and training at:
www.facebook.com/groups/vickiegouldcoaching

Visit her at www.vickiegould.com

Instagram https://www.instagram.com/vickiegould/
Linkedin https://www.linkedin.com/in/vickiegould/
Twitter https://twitter.com/vickie_gould
Facebook page: www.facebook.com/vickiegouldcoach

Made in the USA
Middletown, DE
18 October 2021

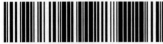